What read

"This is an amazing book by an amazing woman, both truly one of a kind. Janet McBride has gone where no others have ever gone before and has discovered new dimensions in Scriptures that ring true and apply to us today. By her diligent research she has reconciled the wisdom of the ancients with those of modern-day prophets, the energy-wellness movement and 21st century science. Focusing on essential oils and the healing arts as found in the Old and New Testaments, she finds that truly, **"There is nothing new under the sun."** (Eccl. 1:9-10) I was fascinated by her findings of Biblical references to the *chakras*, kinesiology and reflexology. She establishes a solid Scriptural basis for women building home-based businesses through Networking. Her work also reveals two aromatic oils of Scripture heretofore unrecognized as Biblical: Scarlet Root and Lavender — the latter of which she found to have been mentioned 25 times by a Hebrew name never before understood. Thank you, Janet, for your years of scholarship and devotion in compiling this work, doing what no other before you has ever done. This is a resource I will recommend and use in my classes on the spiritual aspects of aromatherapy."

David Stewart PhD, DNM,
President, Center for Aromatherapy Research and Education (CARE), Author of "Healing Oils of the Bible," and other works.
www.raindroptraining.com

"I have practiced Applied Kinesiology for ten years. Janet McBride introduced me to therapeutic grade essential oils and her book, *Scriptural Essence*, and my practice has never been the same since. Her insights have inspired me as I work and research in uncovering many gems of truth found hidden in the meridian system of the human body. Her correlations in applying ancient Hebrew wisdom and the application of essential oils to our modern dilemmas is noteworthy and crucial for the times in which we live."

Carl Skouson Freestone, D.C.
www.doctorfreestone.com

"Scriptural Essence –Temple Secrets Revealed by Rev. Janet McBride is a breath of fresh air. Far too long certain words have frightened the Believer in God—Words like *Chakra* were thought to belong exclusively to the New Age Movement. However, when one knows their Biblical roots and true meanings, they find these gifts are of God, Who is the Author of all things good! Therapeutic Grade Essential Oils are the wave of the future, which God gave to heal His people (Revelation 22:2). Why not get in on that healing wave now and learn about Biblical Essential Oils and their benefits? I for one never travel without Therapeutic Grade **Hyssop, Frankincense** and my own blend, which I call **Isaiah 53 Blend**, made from Therapeutic Grade Essential Oils. I carry the oils in my purse, and it's like carrying pure gold for me. Applying them to my pulse points daily and diffusing them in my home has elevated my mind and spirit. I would not want to be without them!"

Rev. Dr. Barbara A. Di Gilio, ThD,
Founder and President, Mayim Hayim Ministries,
www.mayimhayim.org

Scriptural Essence

**Ancient Temple Secrets Bring
Powerful Healing for Today!**

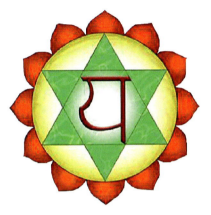

*Heart Chakra in Sanskrit Depicts Star of David
with Pre-Babylonian Hebrew Dalet*

"That which has been is what will be,
That which is done is what will be done,
And there is Nothing New Under the Sun…
<u>It has already been in ancient times before us</u>."

~ Ecclesiastes 1:9-10

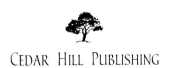

CEDAR HILL PUBLISHING

Scriptural Essence© 2001, 2006
Revised 5th Edition 2006

All Rights Reserved by the McBride Family Trust

Cover design by Rebecca Hayes

Book design by Rebecca Hayes

Published in the United States by

ISBN-10: 1-933324-59-7
ISBN-13: 978-1-933324-59-3

Library of Congress Control Number 2006936517

Acknowledgments

The finished product of **Scriptural Essence**, **Temple Secrets Revealed,** would not be possible without a treasure trove of talent, skill, wisdom, love and unity. I want to especially acknowledge just a few…

Dr. Leonard G. Horowitz, a prolific writer and inspired champion for truth, who fearlessly labors to expose the spiritual wickedness in high places. Dr. Horowitz brings **Healing Celebrations** to a world that seeks a more excellent way.

D. Gary Young, N.D., whose commitment and passion to restore the power of Biblical Essential Oils has taken Health and Wellness to a new level. You are God's Earthly Representative for true Aromatherapy.

Dr. David Stewart PhD, DNM, whose humility, inspiration and *Agape* love for his fellow man has blazed a trail for others to follow in the realm of natural healing…body, soul and spirit.

Rev. Barbara A. Di Gilio ThD, Founder and President of *Mayim-Hayim Ministries,* for her tireless efforts to help restore the Hebraic Truths of the Scriptures to all Believers. I have learned much sitting by her side, gleaning her Gift of Wisdom.

Kitty Robinson, a gifted and committed high school teacher whose talent for critique is incalculable. Thanks for being the Guardian Angel over my many re-writes and edits.

Becky Hayes of Cedar Hill Publishing—Thank you for your abiding patience in my continual "polishing" of the Manuscript and your professional expertise—You made it happen for me!

To My Beloved Joe, the man in whom there is no guile. Thank you for 30 years of love, encouragement, support and belief in my many projects. Thank you for being the Man of Proverbs 31 who sits in the Gates and wisely counsels the younger — especially our children and grandchildren! God's love flows through you, and I am the grateful recipient.

Above all, to **my Divine Healer, Savior and Messiah Yeshua**. Therapeutic Grade Essential Oils are His healing balm, and He alone gets the glory for quickening to our understanding, the Gift of Oils for Health and Wellness in these End Times. Once again, the "Balm of Gilead" is available to all who have an open mind and loving heart. May you *"Be in Health and Prosper, even as your Soul Prospers."* 3rd *John 2*

— Rev. Janet McBride

Table of Contents

Preface 1

Introduction 2

The Original Medicine 3

Temple Secrets Revealed 5
    CHAKRAS IN THE TEMPLE 11
    THE TEMPLE MATRIX 14
    BIBLICAL KINESIOLOGY 16

Sorcery Or Solutions? 18

All Roads Do Not Lead to Health! 18

Scriptural Essence ... The Power to Heal 22
    SANCTIFIED and ANOINTED FEET 22
    Mosaic Healing Laws 23
    Auricular and VitaFlex Charts 24
    THE OILS OF ANCIENT SCRIPTURE 25
    HYSSOP – *Esob* (Holy Herb) 26
    CEDARWOOD – *Erez* (From Root Strength) 27
    MYRTLE – *Hadassah* (From the Tree) 27
    MYRRH – *Mowr* (More Bitter) 29
    FRANKINCENSE *Levonah* (From Tree Resin) ... 30
    GALBANUM *Cheleb* (The Fat) 31
    ALOES-SANDALWOOD *Ahaliym* (Wood Sticks) ... 32
    CASSIA - *Qadad* (Bow the Head) 33
    CYPRESS - *Tirzah* (Slender) 34
    ONYCHA -- *Shecheleth* (Aromatic Shell) 36
    ROSE OF SHARON-CISTUS – *Chaba tstseleth* (Meadow Saffron) 37
    SPIKENARD - *Nard* (Earthy Fragrant Plant) 38
    PINE – *Tid-Har* (Enduring, Lasting) 39
    FIR– *Ber-osh* (A Lance or Musical Instrument) .. 40
    BALSAM FIR - *Tsor'iy* (Balm, Healing Ointment) .. 42

CALAMUS – *Qaneh* (Measuring Reed or a Balance) 43
PEPPERMINT – *Heduosmon* (Gladness, Sweet Scent) 44
ANISE – *Anethon* (of the Dill) 45
CUMIN – *Kammon* (To Store Up, Preserve) 46
MIRACLE OF EGYPTIAN GOLD 47
Egyptian Gold Oil Blend 48
The Pomegranate And The Oils 48

Proverbs 31 Virtuous Businesswoman 51

The Miracle of the Unseen Hand 66
THE MIRACLES BEGIN 68

The Vision of War 71

A Final Thought… 73

About the Author

Janet McBride

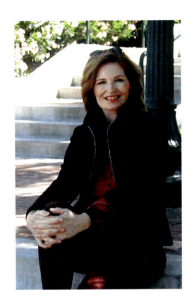

Psalmist, Author, Radio Talk Show Personality, Ordained Minister, Businesswoman and Teacher of Hebraic Studies.

Janet McBride has been a student of Hebraic Roots for more than a decade. As a career military wife, she lived all over the world and came to appreciate the unique gifts of many different cultures. In 1996, Janet left the Corporate World as an Engineering Administrator to open the **House of Judah,** a Hebraic Bookstore in Phoenix, Arizona. She has appeared on numerous radio talk shows discussing the Secrets of Biblical Health.

Janet is following her passion to bring a message of hope to a hurting world through the healing power of Therapeutic Essential Oils. Ordained in 2003 to minister with *Mayim Hayim Ministries*, she embraces total healing of the body, soul and spirit through prayer and Essential Oils. Janet is also a Psalmist and has written over 50 songs.

As a successful business executive, Janet has been featured in ***Who's Who of American Women*** every year since 2002. She launched the ***Virtuous Woman Experience*** to showcase God's original plan for Women to combine a successful home-based business with the higher calling of *Minister of the Home.* Janet teaches that the virtuous women of the Bible were a Positive Force in their Communities, according to the Original Hebrew Language of Proverbs 31. ***"If Health and Prosperity are to become the Biblical Standard in the Home, the Proverbs 31 Woman is the catalyst to bring it to fruition."*** *– Janet McBride*

Preface

This discussion of essential oils and natural scents as depicted in the *Holy Bible* is taken from the original Hebrew and Greek languages, the *Talmud,* the *Apochrypha* and other Ancient religious and historical texts.

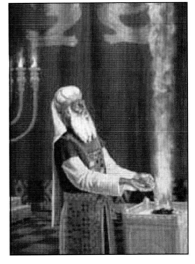

A veil of mystery concealed the Art of Biblical Aromatherapy for centuries. Only the very rich and powerful had access or knowledge of essential oils—And even this knowledge and expertise was virtually lost during the Dark Ages.

With the 20th Century came the so-called "wonder drugs" and a trillion dollar industry of pharmaceutical prescriptions. Any suggestion of modern-day Aromatherapy was labeled Sorcery, Metaphysical or *New Age*.

But now, with the inception of Quantum Physics, DNA and Electro-Magnetic Frequency (EMF) Research, coupled with the rediscovery of Therapeutic Grade Essential Oils, these ancient secrets are emerging as the most powerful natural healing venues of the 21st Century.

It is this author's belief that all that is needed for life, liberty, security, wealth and peace of mind is contained within the pages of the original language of Scripture. It's time to take off the veil, open your eyes and "Let God out of the Box" of religion and tradition. So let us begin, because this is the time of **New Beginnings**.

Introduction

The power and mystique of fragrance has captured the imagination of both men and women for centuries. Spices and oils were an integral part of the religious and health cultures of Biblical times, used in priestly rituals and for anointing the worship instruments in the Temple. The implementation of Therapeutic Grade Essential Oils was the ideal practice employed by the most prominent households.

Essential oils truly are the **Missing Link To Modern Medicine.** The Bible records the occurrence and application of essential oils in over 200 references. They were diffused in the Temple; applied to the sick; given as the **Tithe**; and most likely, one of the many tools employed by the Proverbs 31 Businesswoman.

The concept of the Biblical Home-Based Business is being embraced by the *Baby Boomer* generation looking to improve overall health and wellness and escape the stress of the Corporate Rat Race. Women especially are seeking viable avenues to enable them to work from home to protect and instruct their children in a nurtured environment.

Together, let us embrace the Ancient Temple Secrets and experience the Abundant Life that God promises to His children. You are invited to journey with me into the past to discover your pathway to a healthy and prosperous future. Regardless of your age, background, gender or present circumstances, there is room for you on this 21st Century "Yellow Brick Road." How do you know that you have not been born except for such a time as this? No need to die with the music still inside… Take a deep breath and stop to smell the roses… For truly, **the Path to Wellness is Paved with "Common Scents."**

The Original Medicine

Essential oils were God's original medicine, created on the Third Day. Before Adam was, there were essential oils, and the *"Spirit of God 'Vibrated' over the face of the waters,"*(Genesis 1:2) infusing all creation with the *Frequency* of the Creator:

"And the earth brought forth grass, the herb that yields seed according to its kind, and the tree that yields fruit, whose seed is in itself according to its kind. And God saw that it was good. So the evening and the morning were the Third Day." (*Gen 1:13*)

Essential oils are the lifeblood of every tree, plant, leaf and herb. The oil of the plant is nearly 50 times more potent in therapeutic content than the dried herb or flower. The application of therapeutic grade essential oils transforms *dis-eased* (a body imbalance) tissue into thriving, healthy cells.

During the Mosaic Period, special oils were designated by God to sanctify (set apart) an entire Hebraic genealogy known as the *Cohanim* (priests). The ritual anointing of these priests distinguished them not only for Temple service; but according to Rabbi Aryeh Kaplan's scholarly theory of the *Torah* (Exodus 40:1, 12-16), this anointing and separation actually registered in the DNA of their cells and continues throughout their generations.* And today, technology proves the existence of a distinctive Y-chromosome in the DNA of Aaron's descendants. **

*The Living Torah, 1982
** Science News, Oct 3, 1998

Just as the Levitical priests received a holy anointing, the Scriptures tell us that special anointings were also designated to treat *dis-eases* like Leprosy and to release emotional patterns of Guilt. (Leviticus 14:28-29)

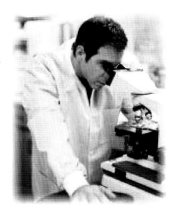

While it is unlikely the priests of ancient Israel fully understood the significance of these applications, contemporary research is confirming that these applications can — AND DO — effect dramatic healing in the body, the mind and even the spirit. The ancient secrets of the Temple priests have emerged as powerful tools to heal the body, our Temples.

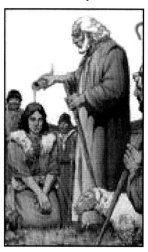

"And the Lord said to Moses, 'You shall bring Aaron and his sons to the door of the Tabernacle of meeting, and you shall…take the **anointing oil**, pour it on the head and **anoint** them.'"

~ *Exodus 29:4-8*

Temple Secrets Revealed

What were the Ancient Secrets given to Moses and Aaron? Was there a mysterious and miraculous healing power imparted through the application of essential oils? Did King Solomon have a unique understanding of how oils could release emotion and passion when he wrote the *"Song of Songs"* to his Beloved? Why were essential oils consistently used on the Messiah Yeshua (Jesus Christ)? And what was the secret of duplication and networking employed by the Proverbs 31 woman? Science and Scripture give us clues to unlocking these and many more secrets behind longevity with vitality, unlimited wealth and prosperity, and the Art of Biblical Aromatherapy:

Secret No. 1 – Research and technology of the latter 20th Century confirm that a healthy human body registers an electrical frequency between 62 and 68 MHz (Mega Hertz). *Dis-ease*, which is a body imbalance, begins when the body's frequency drops below 58 MHz. Therapeutic grade essential oils are alive with natural frequencies of their own which act upon the human body to stimulate, energize and enhance frequency levels. [Taino Technology, 1992]

Secret No. 2 – Therapeutic grade essential oils contain constituents such as sesquiterpenes, proven to bypass the blood-brain barrier. They actually pass through the region of the brain called the Amygdala, which allows their healing properties to penetrate remote areas of the brain that are inaccessible through surgery or drugs. Sesquiterpenes also promote the natural release of Human Growth Hormones and other vital hormones such as Serotonin to defend against depression. Several high-sesquiterpene oils are mentioned by name throughout the pages of Scripture: **Frankincense, Cedarwood** and **Aloes-Sandalwood**.

Secret No. 3 – Most viruses, fungi and bacteria cannot sustain themselves in the presence of therapeutic grade essential oils. Moses directed the children of Israel to dip **Hyssop** branches into the blood and strike the doorposts to protect against the deadly plague. Hyssop is a highly anti-bacterial, anti-viral essential oil. *(Exodus 12:22)*

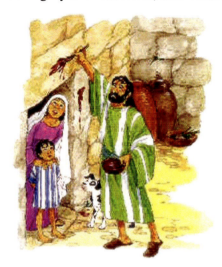

Centuries later, during the infamous Black Plague of the 14th century, a group of bandits robbed its victims without succumbing to the mysterious virus. When questioned under penalty of death, they confessed that a blend of essential oils protected them from the deadly Plague. Through careful control of the growth and distillation process, Young Living Essential Oils has closely duplicated this recipe.*

Secret No. 4 – The human body contains more than 1,400 VitaFlex points. The soles of the feet are mirror images of the internal workings of these points of energy. The Lord God of Israel sanctified the feet of the priests and told Joshua that as soon as the ***soles of the feet*** of those who bore the Ark of the Covenant (e.g., the priests) touched the waters of the Jordan…indeed they would divide and stand as a heap.** … And so it was. Research has found that careful application of therapeutic essential oils to the soles of the feet enables the oil to reach every cell in the body within 20 minutes.***

* *Essential Oils Desk Ref, 1st Ed, Ess. Sci Pub, pg. 48*
** *Joshua 3:13*
*** *Introduction to Essential Oils, 9th Edition, Pg. 20*

"And the Lord God...<u>Breathed into his Nostrils</u> the Breath of Life..."' (Gen. 2:7)

Secret No. 5 – Essential Oils, through **Inhalation** of their aromas, can directly stimulate the limbic region of the brain and exert a profound effect on the body and the mind. Inhaling or **"breathing-in"** is facilitated through the olfactory nerve and invites the oils' constituents into these regions of the brain. This enables the body to process them naturally. It is widely held that essential oils can effect mood changes, spiritual clarity and physical stimulation. Even the Creator was moved to compassion through inhalation of a sweet-smelling sacrifice following the flood:

"Then Noah built an altar to God and offered burnt offerings... and the Lord <u>smelled a soothing aroma</u> and said in His heart, 'I will never again curse the ground for man's sake...'" ~ Gen. 8:20-21

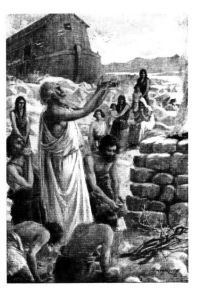

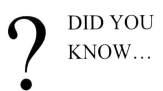 DID YOU KNOW...

That true Inhalation requires that you **Inhale through the Nostrils** and **Exhale through the Mouth?** Most people understand the importance of **smelling** the aromas to benefit from their healing properties. But Inhalation is much more that "sniffing." **Inhaling deeply through the nose** takes in life-giving oxygen from the oils and exhaling through the mouth allows the body to expel harmful toxins. Inhaling through the mouth does not allow detoxification.

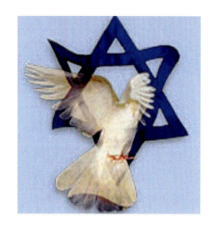

Secret No. 6 – In conjunction with Inhalation is the Sense of **Smell**. Of the five physical senses, Smell is the only one that can effectively heal the emotions. And of even greater significance is the Biblical word for **"smell."** It is identical to the Hebrew word for **"spirit"** – **Ruach**. Thus, the Holy Spirit, e.g., the **Ruach ha Kodesh,** infers by its Hebraic meaning that God's Spirit is accessed through the **sense of smell**. Perhaps this is the reason therapeutic grade essential oils have the potential to unlock and release spiritual trauma**.**

DID YOU KNOW…

?
That in Ancient Biblical times, the Spirit of God was often called the *"Essence of God,"* because *Ruach* means **Smell** as well as **Spirit.**

Science has shown that repressed traumas are actually stored in different organs of the body. This same research has also shown that memories are not only stored in the brain, but in the whole psychosomatic network of the body. This is particularly true of nerve receptors. *(Molecules of Emotion – Dr. Candace Pert)*

King Solomon in ancient times understood the awesome healing power of fragrance and its effect on emotions when he wrote:

"Ointment (oils) and fragrance delight the heart." ~ Proverbs 27:9

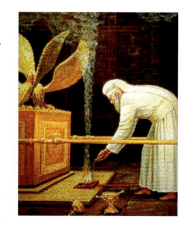

Secret No. 7 – Therapeutic grade essential oils encourage longevity and regeneration of cell tissue. This may shed some light as to why the people in ancient times lived to such advanced age with strength and vigor. Regular inhalation of essential oils stimulates the limbic region of the brain and encourages the natural release of the human growth hormone (HGH). Continued enhancement of the body's vibrational frequency through the use of therapeutic grade essential oils supports greater longevity with optimum health.

Moses and Aaron were repeatedly exposed to the fragrance of the oils because of their priestly duties. And upon his death at the age of 120 years, Scripture tells us that Moses' eyesight was still excellent and his natural energy still vibrant:

"Moses was one hundred and twenty years old when he died. His eyes were not dimmed, and his vigor had not diminished."
~ Deut. 34:7

There are still remote cultures in the world today where longevity with vitality is the norm, rather than the exception. The Hunza people in Northern Pakistan; the Province of Ningxia in Northern China; and the Talish Mountains of Azerbaijan. The common denominators in these communities seem to be an active lifestyle, combined with a mineral-rich diet, exceptionally high in antioxidant foods. *

---

* Essential Oils Desk Reference, 3rd Edition, p. 266

Secret No. 8 – The Human Body is actually a Sacred Temple that houses the *Essence* of the Creator:

"Do you not know that you are the Temple of the Holy Spirit (Essence of God), Who lives in you? If anyone <u>Defiles the Temple</u>, he will be ***phtheiro*** *[Greek for Wasted and Lose Strength]. For the Temple of God is holy, <u>which Temple you are</u>." ~ 1st Corinthians 3:16-17*

If the human body is, as the Bible says, a Temple for the Spirit or the *Essence* of God, then we must understand ***our <u>responsibility</u> to care for it*** and observe what we put in it and on it. If we defile it, the result is a wasting away of the body and loss of strength, i.e., ability to fight *dis-ease*. It's not a matter of being "under the law" or "free from the law." It's a matter of **Universal Natural Law** that, like Gravity, has a built-in <u>Cause and Effect</u>. Free Will gives us a choice, but choices have consequences.

Secret No. 9 – Everything in Creation vibrates with the <u>frequency</u> of the Creator. This includes the essential oils that are extracted from the plant kingdom. These plant oils are organically compatible with the human body, which also vibrates with that same frequency. When harvested and distilled at the *Therapeutic Grade Level*, the oils have no adverse side effects. How does this happen? The secret is recorded in the original Hebrew of Genesis:

"The Spirit of God <u>Vibrated</u> (Ra'chaph) on the face of the waters."
~ Genesis 1;2

Consequently, all creation vibrates with the measurable frequency of the *Essence of God*

Secret No. 10 – Within our physical Temple structure, there is a beautiful picture of the *Menorah,* the Lampstand of God. In the original Temple design, God commanded a *Menorah* of pure gold be set within the Temple and its light was to never go out. (Lev. 24:3)

The description of the *Menorah* is a mirror image of the seven electrical energy centers of the spinal column, known as *Chakras*. These energy points transport the body's electrical frequency through the spine to nourish and strengthen the body systems. The seven *chakras* represent the Seven-Lamp *Menorah* of our Temples, transmitting the life-giving Light of God's Spirit.

The Ancient *Menorah* had seven lamps, and a center shaft, or **"Heart,"** which coincides with the centermost point of the seven *chakras* of the Spine. There are three *Chakras* on either side of the **"Heart"** *Chakra*, similar to the Temple *Menorah*:

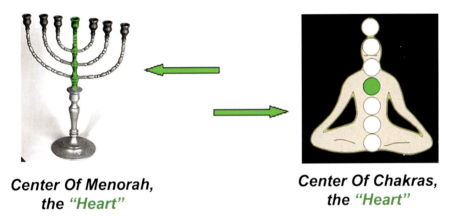

Center Of Menorah, the "Heart"

Center Of Chakras, the "Heart"

*"The Menorah shall be of one piece and so, too, its shaft (**Heart**), and three branches on one side and three branches on the other side."*
~ Exodus 25:31-32

CHAKRAS IN THE TEMPLE

The Word **"Chakra"** is a Sanskrit word from an ancient sacred language meaning a **"Wheel."** After God confused the language of the Earth at the building of the Tower of Babel (*Genesis Chapter 11*), each new language still retained remnants of the original unified Earth language. And to this day you can find similarities in all

Semitic and Ancient languages. These include Hebrew and Greek, the original languages of the Bible.

God commanded the *Menorah* of the Temple to be tended daily, and that oils and incense be diffused on it during the process. So, too, the *Chakras* need regular attention lest there be an energy block in the spine, resulting in pain, dysfunction and *dis-ease*. Similar to the ancient practice of employing fragrance to light the *Menorah*, the best way to light-up the *Chakras* is by the strategic application of essential oils:

"And when Aaron lights the Menorah in the morning and at twilight, he shall diffuse on it Sweet Frankincense, a perpetual incense before the Lord throughout your generations."
~ Exodus 30: 7-8

"...And in the Middle (Heart) of the 7 Menorahs Stands One like the Son of Man (Yeshua).."
~ Revelation 1:13

? DID YOU KNOW…

● The ancient symbol for the **Heart Chakra**, the ***Center Shaft of the Body's Menorah***, is depicted with the Pre-Babylonian Hebrew Letter "**D**" called ***Dalet***. Not only that, but this Hebrew Letter is encased in a **Star of David**. This is an example of how the ancient languages all contain remnants of the original Earth language. In the original Hebrew language, the ***Dalet*** **(D)** is called ***"The Door"*** *and* was written in this way:

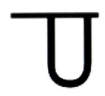 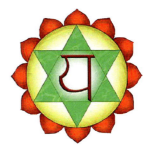

Original 4th Letter of Hebrew - *The Door* *

Ancient Symbol for the Heart (Center) 4th Chakra

* Hebrew Word Dictionary – Frank Seekins

When the word "Door" appears in Scripture, its literal meaning is "Portal" or "Gateway." Likewise, the *Heart Chakra* is the "Gateway" to the other six energy centers of the body. The three below the *Heart Chakra* affect the emotions and the physical body. This is how we're grounded to the Earth. The three above the *Heart Chakra* affect the mind and the spirit. This is our mental-spiritual connection to the Creator.

Is it just a coincidence that the *Heart Chakra*, the Gateway, is the 4th *Chakra;* and the *Dalet,* the **"Door"** is the fourth letter of the Hebrew Alphabet? Scripture tells us **"The Door"** is a Person:

"I am the Door. If anyone enters by Me, he will be saved and will go in and out…" ~ Words of Yeshua (John 10:9)

This Author believes the Hebrew Symbol for the *Heart Chakra* is the same Sacred Symbol described by the Prophet Ezekial in his Vision of the "Wheel Within a Wheel" (Chakra within a Chakra):

- Appeared to have the color of **Beryl Stone** – *(Ezekial 1:16)*
- NOTE: A **Beryl Stone** was Over the Heart Chakra on the Priest's Breastplate *(Exodus 28:20)*
- They were called "Wheels" (Chakras) *(Ezekial 10:13)*
- The Wheels were full of eyes *(Ezekial 1:18)*
- The rim of the wheel had "eyes" all around *(Ezekial 10:12)*

THE TEMPLE MATRIX

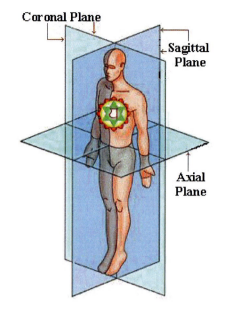

A *Matrix* is defined among other things as *"A rectangular array of numerical quantities… A Network of Intersections between "input" and "output," as in a computer… A womb in which something originates, develops or is contained."* (American Heritage Dictionary, 2nd College Edition)

Remarkably, the Ancient Scriptures speak of a **Matrix** within the Earthly Temple known as the *"Heart"* or the *"Belly"* of man." *(Strong's Exhaustive Concordance, Nelson Publishers)*

The Hebrew word for Matrix is *Me'ah* and is found in **Psalm 40:8**: "Yea, Thy Law is Within my *Matrix.*"

The Greek word for Matrix is *Koilia* and is found in **John 7:38**:

"He that Believes in Me, as the Scripture has said, 'Out of his Matrix Shall Flow Rivers of Living Water.'"
-- (Words of Yeshua)

The Universal Laws of Creation are woven within the Body's *Matrix* and work autonomously with no effort on our part. This *Matrix* is a Network of Portals, Gateways and Meridian Points through which passes DNA information, vibrational frequency, emotional experiences, and spiritual communiqués.

The *Matrix* includes the Electrical Meridian Pathways used in Traditional Chinese Medicine (TCM). The ancient art of Acupuncture is based on the Temple's intricate network of electrical channels that run throughout the entire structure. Practitioners believe that imbalances in the natural flow of energy through this *Matrix* result in *dis-ease.*

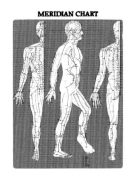

Interestingly, in keeping with the model of the Ancient Temple design, the *Matrix* in the human body consists of 12 Meridians. Likewise, there are 12 Tribes of Israel; 12 Gates to the City of Jerusalem; 12 Months on the ancient and modern-day calendars; 12 Crystals on the Breastplate of the Temple High Priest; 12 Gates to the walls of the New Jerusalem; 12 Trees that grow along the Crystal Sea, etc.

The 12 Meridians are divided into six <u>Positive</u> and six <u>Negative</u> Frequency channels. Like all magnetic patterns, the Meridians fully support the *Polarity* of the body's flow of natural energy. And like the *Chakras*, it is prudent to keep these Temple pathways clear of harmful influences.

The Temple *Matrix* is also defined in the Greek as a womb* where life originates. It is in this part of the *Matrix* where viruses, bacteria and other *dis-eases* take root and grow. Therapeutic grade essential oils help to clear the Temple *Matrix* of blocked passageways, rid the system of bacteria, and promote healing throughout the entire Temple—body, soul and spirit.

* *Strong's Exhaustive Concordance, Nelson Publishers*

BIBLICAL KINESIOLOGY

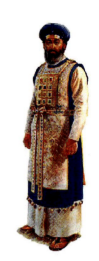

Applied Kinesiology (AK) is a science that uses muscle testing as a diagnostic tool for the health of the body. When properly applied, the outcome of an AK diagnosis will determine the best form of therapy for the patient. In ancient times, a similar form of diagnostics or Temple inquiry was achieved through a mysterious vibrational frequency emanating from the crystalline breastplate of the Temple High Priest. Scriptures tell us this mysterious vibration called ***Urim*** and ***Thummin*** occurred when certain gemstones embedded in the breastplate were illuminated by the Vibration of God's Essence. The High Priest would then make inquiry for guidance, judgments and prophecy. *(Levit. 28:30)*

The Hebrew word ***Urim*** means *"to kindle, to light a fire."* In keeping with the placement of the ***Urim*** on the breastplate, this would have likely been right over the *Heart Chakra*, the Center Stem of the Body's *Menorah*. In Hebrew tradition when lighting a *Menorah*, the fire of the Center Lamp, the *Heart*, is kindled first. Then all other lamps are lit from the *Heart* of the *Menorah*.

The ***Thummin***, also placed strategically over the *Heart Chakra,* means ***"Perfect Truth."*** The modern day Science of Kinesiology has proven that the body does not lie! Dr. John Diamond's work in Behavioral Kinesiology (*Your Body Doesn't Lie – John Diamond, M.D.)* reveals the Thymus Gland, a Kinetic indicator for the body, is actually a barometer for ***"Truth."*** The end of the Thymus is coincidentally located at the *Heart Chakra.* The body, through Kinetic testing, communicates what it needs at any given moment. It can test the vibrational frequency of essential oils against the body's frequency. And we know this Kinetic ability comes from God:

"For in Him we live and* MOVE *(Greek word KINEO) and have our being..." ~ Acts 17:28

So how does this God-given Kinesiology work? We must take our cue from the Scriptures. Whenever we see a record of the Glory of God manifesting, the people fell on their faces—that is, they fell *"forward."* But, when a negative energy approached, those entities would fall or be driven *"backward."* Negativity cannot stand in the presence of God's Spirit. But positive energy expresses **humility** in God's presence.

"When the priests and the people standing in the courtyard knew that the Name of the Lord was pronounced they bowed [forward], prostrated themselves, gave thanks, **fell to their faces** and said, 'Blessed is the Name and the honor of His kingdom forever and ever.'" ~ **The Yom Kippur Machzor***

Likewise, when the **Shekinah Glory** filled the Temple, the priests were overcome and could not stand.** Conversely, when Messiah Yeshua was about to be arrested in the Garden of Gethsemane, the negative energy of His captors' intentions caused them to *fall "backwards"* when He spoke His Name, **"I AM."** ***

So our Biblical Guidance to test Essential Oils is with our Temple's Kinetic Indicator, the **Heart Chakra**. Hold the Essential Oil against the 4th *Chakra* at the end of the Thymus Gland. Close your eyes; say nothing. Experience the frequency of the Oil in response to your Temple's frequency. If the Oil is needed, you will feel yourself gently falling **"forward"** into the frequency of that oil. If you do not need it, you will gently feel yourself falling "backward," away from the frequency. No movement indicates the Oil is Neutral to you.

*   2nd Chronicles 29:29
** 1st Kings 8:10-11
*** John 18: 5-6

Sorcery Or Solutions?
All Roads Do Not Lead to Health!

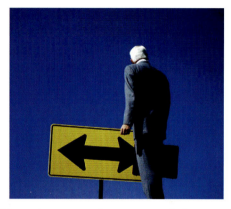

***"There is a way that seems right to man,
but its end is the way of Death."***
~ (Proverbs 14:12)

When it comes to the subject of Medicine, the Bible gives very specific guidelines: Essential oils, spices, herbs, grasses, and ointments are **in harmony with Nature.** That same vibrational frequency that was infused into the *"Dust of the Earth"* at the time of Creation continues to fuel the life force of all living things. *(Genesis 2:7)*

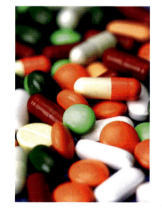

In stark contrast, the so-called Designer Drugs of the 21st Century are merely synthetic, toxic imitations of God's Original Medicine.

Since essential oils, herbs and grasses cannot be patented, it was deemed necessary to create controlled substances that are very predictable. Hence, the birth of prescription drugs! In conjunction with these man-made synthetics came serum injections called **"Vaccines."** In a time when serious illness was in epidemic proportions, these so-called "Wonder Drugs" gained huge acceptance; and today, these are the only medicines endorsed by the American Medical Association, University Medical Schools, and the Food and Drug Administration (FDA).

As a result, we now have mutating Super Bugs, Fibromyalgia, Chronic Fatigue Syndrome, environmental and chemical sensitivities, while Autism, ADD and Morbid Obesity are reaching epidemic levels. The devastating side effects from these synthetic drugs and LIVE Virus Vaccines have made the ancient Biblical warning of **"Defiling the Temple"** a stark reality! And the wisdom of King Solomon now overshadows the whole Earth:

"There is a way that seems right to man, but its end is the way of Death." ~ Proverbs 14:12

? DID YOU KNOW…

The Scriptures foretold a day when Sorcery and Witchcraft would appear in the form of pharmaceutical drugs?

"Now the Works of the Flesh are evident… SORCERY, of which I tell you beforehand… those who practice such things will not inherit the Kingdom of God." ~ Galatians 5:20

The word "Sorcery" in this passage presents us with a new definition in the original language of Scripture:

Greek Word **Pharmakeia** – Medicine, pharmacy, sorcery, witchcraft (*Pharmaceuticals*)

> *"And they did not repent of their murders and their <u>sorceries</u>…" (Pharmaceuticals) ~ Revelation 9:21*

> *"…For by your <u>sorcery</u>, all the nations were deceived." (Pharmaceuticals) ~ Revelation 21:8*

CONTRAST THIS SORCERY WITH GOD'S SOLUTION FOR HEALING:

*"…All kinds of trees grow…Their leaves will be for **medicine**." (Ezekial 47:12)* Medicine in this verse is the Hebrew word **Rapha,** which means a **remedy**, to **heal**, to **cure**, to **make whole**.

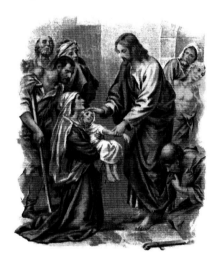

"And they cast out many demons and <u>anointed with oil</u> many who were sick <u>and healed them</u>." ~ Mark 6:13

"A certain Samaritan… had compassion on him and bandaged his wounds, <u>pouring on oil</u>…" ~ Luke 10:33-34

"Is any sick among you? Let him call for the Elders of the Church and let them pray over him, <u>anointing him with oil</u> in the Name of the Lord." ~ James 5:14

During the first century Common Era (CE), the Elders were versed in the customs of the day, which included the application and use of essential oils for healing. The oil used in the anointing of the sick was an essential oil applied to the body in accordance with the Holy Scriptures (Leviticus 14:17, for example). And this knowledge is the birthright of the Believers in the 21st century.

But sadly, most Christians today mistakenly believe that the *physicians* mentioned in Scripture were the same as our contemporary medical doctors—**not so**! Today's licensed Medical Doctors (MDs), though well intentioned, are not educated in the healing arts of old — rather, they are experts in the art of prescribing **pharmaceuticals** and performing invasive diagnostic procedures and surgeries. Conversely, the Biblical physician actually <u>cured</u> *dis-ease*. In Hebrew, the word for physician is *Rapha;* in Greek the word is *Iasis* – Both defined as **healer, one who makes whole, cures**. *(Strong's Exhaustive Concordance, Nelson Publishers)*

"Luke, the beloved physician greets you." -- *Colossians 4:14*

Scriptural Essence ...
The Power to Heal

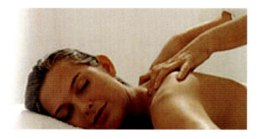
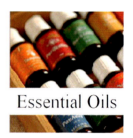

Essential Oils

"Beloved, I Pray that You may Prosper in all things and Be in Health, Just as your Soul Prospers."
~ *3rd John 2*

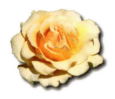

SANCTIFIED and ANOINTED FEET

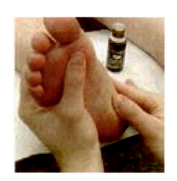

As mentioned in Ancient Secret No. 4, anointing the ***"soles of the feet"*** with essential oil enables you to directly influence the VitaFlex points connected to every body system. In the following Scripture passage, Mary of Bethany anointed the ***feet*** of the Messiah Yeshua in this way:

> *"They made Him a supper... and sat at the table with Him.
> Then Mary (sister of Lazarus) took a pound of very costly
> Oil of Spikenard, anointed the feet of Jesus,
> and wiped His feet with her hair." (John 12:3)*

On another occasion, a woman of questionable reputation anointed the feet of Messiah Yeshua. In her act of humility and repentance, she wept over his feet, washing them with her hair and then anointing Him with essential oil:

> *"...And she began to wash His feet with her tears, and wiped them with the hair of her head; and she kissed His feet and anointed them with the fragrant oil." ~ Luke 7:38*

Mosaic Healing Laws

The ancient rituals of *Torah* also required the use of essential oils for cleansing Leprosy and absolving Guilt. The oils of Hyssop, Scarlet and Cedarwood were defined as part of these rituals. God commanded the priest to anoint the Leper in the same manner as the Guilt offering, which was to anoint the top of the right ear, the thumb of the right hand, and the big toe on the right foot. (*Leviticus 14:17*) These are the specific VitaFlex points for the Limbic region of the brain, located in your "Temple" as shown by scientific research. (*Essential Oils Desk Reference, 3rd Edition*)

Auricular and VitaFlex Charts

According to the Auricular Emotions Chart,* the top of the right ear is the VitaFlex point to release Guilt. The thumb on the right hand and the big toe on the right foot are the VitaFlex points for the Brain and Pineal gland — the center of the body's communication system and the place where emotional memory is stored.**

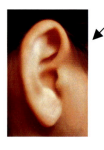

Releasing Guilt on Auricular Chart
"And the priest shall put some of the oil that is in his hand on the tip of the right ear of him who is to be cleansed... on the place of the guilt offering."
~ Leviticus 14:17

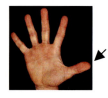

Brain and Pituitary Point on VitaFlex Chart
"And the priest shall put some of the oil that is in his hand on... the thumb of the right hand..."
~ Leviticus 14:17

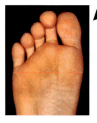

Brain and Pituitary Point on VitaFlex Chart
"And the priest shall put some of the oil that is in his hand on... the big toe of the right foot."
~ Leviticus 14:17

* *Essential Oils Desk Reference, 1st Edition, p. 181*
** *Essential Oils Desk Reference, 1st Edition, p. 173*

The essential oils of ***Cedarwood, Scarlet and Hyssop*** are used for specific therapeutic techniques—both physically and emotionally. Psalm 51:7 says, *"Purge me with hyssop and I shall be clean..."* (Free from Guilt).

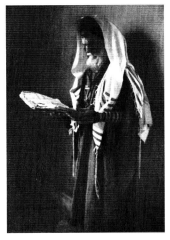

The English translation of the word, "scarlet" in the *Torah* is, in my opinion, an incorrect translation. The original Hebrew text carries no Hebraic rendering of the word, "scarlet."

However, since the Lord directed Moses to use two other natural substances containing therapeutic essential oils, i.e.: Cedarwood and Hyssop, we can logically expect that the word *Scarlet* inserted into this Levitical passage is not a Scarlet thread or type of material, but actually a Scarlet <u>root</u> that also produces an essential oil. Scarlet root was used extensively in the Middle East in ancient times as a medicinal herb for skin conditions and is believed to have been brought to the Western World by Christopher Columbus. (*The History of Fragrance, Aromatherapy: A Complete Guide to the Healing Art - Crossing Press, **1995***)

THE OILS OF ANCIENT SCRIPTURE

Let's examine the Oils of Ancient Scripture in light of their Hebraic roots and why therapeutic grade essential oils are the **"Missing Link To Modern Medicine."** *(Young Living Essential Oils, D. Gary Young, ND)*

HYSSOP – *Esob* (Holy Herb)

The essential oil of Hyssop is first mentioned in the *Book of the Exodus*. The Lord told Moses to instruct the children of Israel to *strike* the lintel and doorposts with a bunch of Hyssop dipped in the blood of the lamb. This was the first Passover.

The Hebrew word for "strike" (*na'than*) translates "shoots forth" and actually means to **"Diffuse."** When the Hyssop branch was struck across the doorposts and lintel, the essential oil of the plant spewed forth, diffusing a miraculous protection against plague for that entire household. This passage was prophetically fulfilled at Calvary, when **Hyssop** was offered to Yeshua on the Cross and He became the **Final Passover Lamb**:

"So when Yeshua had received the sour wine with Hyssop, He said, 'It is Finished.'" (John 19:29-30)

Essential Oil of Hyssop is:

a. Anti-asthmatic; anti-infectious; anti-inflammatory; antioxidant; anti-parasitic; antiseptic; antispasmodic; anti-viral; decongestant; diuretic; and sedative. Not for pregnant women.

b. Hyssop can help with coughs, colds and fever, asthma, parasites, regulating lipid metabolism, strengthening and toning the nervous system; help prevent scarring and aid with viral infections.

c. <u>For emotional clearing</u>: Hyssop stimulates the 6th Chakra to clear the mind.* Helps release swallowed emotions and old thought patterns. Heightens ability to focus.**

* *Vibrational Healing with Essential Oils* – D. Eidson
** *Releasing Emotional Patterns with Essential Oils* – Dr. Mein

CEDARWOOD – *Erez* (From Root Strength)

Added to the Hyssop and Scarlet in the "sacred trio" is the essence of the aromatic and treasured **Cedarwood tree**. Cedarwood has long been revered for its use in storing and protecting possessions, clothing and keepsakes from the harsh elements. Cedarwood is also associated with weddings, in that Tradition says the Bride shall have a chest made of Cedarwood to store her treasures until the great wedding feast.

Essential Oil of Cedarwood is:

a. High in sesquiterpenes that bypass the blood-brain barrier (big toe on right foot VitaFlex point for the brain).

b. May be effective against hair loss, tuberculosis, bronchitis, gonorrhea, urinary infections, acne and psoriasis. Helps to reduce hardening of the artery walls and may assist in stimulating the pineal gland to release natural melatonin for deep sleep.

c. For emotional clearing: Stimulates the 6th Chakra, limbic and emotional regions of the brain through inhalation. Massage Cedarwood into the back of the right thumb to dispel "math" anxiety when taking tests.*

MYRTLE – *Hadassah* (From the Tree)

In the days of Queen Esther, it was not an uncommon practice for Persian women to prepare for their wedding by learning to apply essential oils. This course of study often lasted up to one calendar year.

* Dr. David Stewart

❓ DID YOU KNOW?

A little known fact about Queen Esther is the origin of her name. In the original Hebrew, this daughter of Abraham was called **Hadassah.** The English translation for Hadassah is **Myrtle** —Not Esther.

Myrtle was also a treasured herb used in the celebration of the Feast of Tabernacles (*Sukkot – Nehemiah 8:15*). By its very formation in the earth, Myrtle is a picture of the magnified presence of *Adonai Echad* (the Lord is ONE). The Myrtle leaves are clustered in groups of three, but all grow from the same point on the stem.

The Hebrew word *echad* translates as **"ONE, comprised of more than one."** Myrtle is a picture of a Unified God expressed in three Personalities—One stem comprising three blooms. Torah says:

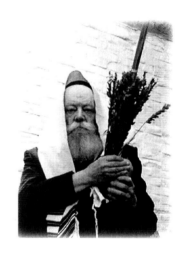

*"Sh'ma Yisra'el! Adonai Eloheinu,
Adonai Echad"*
*"Hear O Israel, the Lord Our God, the
Lord is ONE (Echad)."*
~ Deuteronomy 6:4

Essential Oil of Myrtle is:

a. Anti-infectious; liver stimulant; prostate decongestant; hormone-like properties for thyroid and ovaries; skin tonic.

b. Myrtle can be used to help with asthma, sinus and respiratory infections, tuberculosis and ureter infections. Helps to normalize hormonal imbalances, as well as balance hypothyroidism. *(Dr. Daniel Penoel's Research)*

c. <u>For emotional clearing</u>: Apply Myrtle to the 3rd Chakra to help overcome suppression of the Temple's frequency.* Myrtle helps to balance the Polarity of the Temple Matrix.**

MYRRH – *Mowr* (More Bitter)

Queen Hadassah invested six months of learning to apply the essential oil of Myrrh in preparation for her presentation to the Persian King Ahasuerus as his <u>Bride</u>. And in similar fashion, Myrrh was one of the Treasures presented at the birth of the Messiah <u>Bridegroom</u>. (*Esther 2:12; Matthew 2:11*)

Essential Oil of Myrrh is:

a. Anti-infectious; anti-viral; anti-parasitic; anti-inflammatory; soothes skin conditions; supports immune system; hormonal-like properties. *May be anti-cancer agent per Rutgers University (Journal of Natural Products, November 26, 2001).*

b. Myrrh may help with bronchitis, diarrhea, dysentery, hyperthyroidism, stretch marks, thrush, ulcers, vaginal thrush, viral hepatitis, asthma, athlete's foot, candida, coughs, eczema, digestion, fungal infection, gingivitis, gum infections, hemorrhoids, mouth ulcers, ringworm, sore throats, chapped and cracked skin, wounds and wrinkles.

c. <u>For emotional clearing</u>: Myrrh helps overcome the fear of facing the world when applied to the adrenal alarm points." **

---

*   *Vibrational Healing with Essential Oils* – D. Eidson
** *Releasing Emotional Patterns with Essential Oils* – Dr. Mein

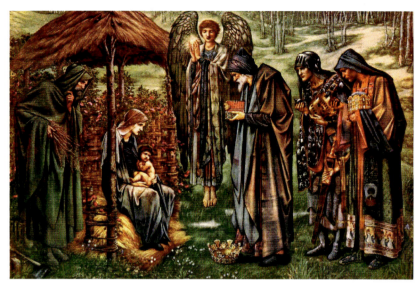

"And They Opened Their Treasures and Offered Him Gifts of [Liquid] Gold, Frankincense **and Myrrh**."
~ *Matthew 2:11*

FRANKINCENSE *Levonah* (From Tree Resin)

The power of Frankincense cannot be captured in one paragraph. Considered by many to be the "holiest of anointing oils," Frankincense has been used by religious cultures worldwide and is included in the sacred recipe applied in the ancient Temple. *

It takes approximately 40 years—one generation in Israel—to grow a Frankincense Tree (Boswellia). Today, research has shown Frankincense is used therapeutically in Europe for its ability to increase HGH (Human Growth Hormone).

"Who is this that cometh out of the Wilderness like pillars of smoke, perfumed with Myrrh and Frankincense…"
~ *Song of Solomon 3:6*

* Exodus 30:34

Essential Oil of Frankincense is:

a. Anti-tumoral, anti-catarrhal and is an immuno-stimulant. It is beneficial in fighting asthma, depression and ulcers. Frankincense increases the activity of leukocytes in defense of the body against infection. It helps with allergies, bites, bronchitis, cancer, Diphtheria, headaches, hemorrhaging, Herpes, hypertension, inflammation, stress, tonsillitis, Typhoid and warts.

b. <u>For emotional clearing</u>: Frankincense is high in sesquiterpenes and can stimulate and elevate the mind to overcome stress and despair (*Essential Oils Desk Reference, 3rd Ed. p54*).

GALBANUM *Cheleb* (The Fat)

There is an interesting suggestion in the Jewish **Talmud** as to why the powerful, less-than-fragrant resin, Galbanum, was used in the holy incense. It represented those needing redemption:

"Every communal fast that does not include the sinners of Israel is not a fast." ~ *Talmud (Keritot 6b)*

This has been linked to the fact that the Temple incense included spices or perfumes with lovely fragrances, BUT was incomplete without one spice — Galbanum, with its earthy aroma. The Hebraic root of Galbanum is *cheleb*, which means "the fat or the richest part." **Torah** teaches that the priest was to offer the goat as an offering made by fire for a sweet aroma, and all the "*cheleb*" (the fat) belonged to the Lord and was forbidden for human consumption (Leviticus 3:14-17). This was — *and still is* — a perpetual statute throughout the generations.

We would do well to adhere to ***Torah's*** warning regarding the fat. America now experiences epidemic stages of morbid obesity and a level of *dis-ease* never before seen due to the amount of fat content in our diets. Sadly, we now have a ***Journal of Pediatric Obesity*** because the incidence of childhood obesity has skyrocketed.

Essential Oil of Galbanum is:

a. Anti-infectious, anti-inflammatory, stimulating, supportive to the kidneys and women's menstrual cycles, analgesic and lightly anti-spasmodic.

b. Galbanum helps combat asthma, inflammation, poor circulation and wounds. It may help with abscesses, acne, bronchitis, cramps, stress, indigestion, muscular aches and pains, nervous tension, rheumatism, scar tissue, and wrinkles.

c. <u>For emotional clearing</u>: Galbanum brings harmony and balance. It may also help to increase spiritual awareness and meditation.

ALOES-SANDALWOOD *Ahaliym* (Wood Sticks)

Many botanists believe that Aloes were derived from Sandalwood. Aloes-Sandalwood is a resin released by the tree to defend against fungus once the tree has fallen. As a result, Aloes-Sandalwood develops very slowly over time – typically SEVERAL HUNDRED YEARS or more. This is why Aloes-Sandalwood is so rare and highly valued, in addition to its wonderful aroma.

Although he initially planned to curse Israel, in the end, the prophet *Balaam* blessed Israel, comparing her to "***Aloes** planted by the Lord.*" (*Numbers 24:6*) This reference suggests that Aloes-

Sandalwood was a planting to be treasured as something *spiritually* unique.

Essential Oil of Aloes-Sandalwood is:

a. Rich in sesquiterpenes like Frankincense and Cedarwood. Aloes-Sandalwood stimulates the Limbic Region of the brain, which is responsible for releasing melatonin, a powerful antioxidant that enhances deep sleep. And like Frankincense, Aloes-Sandalwood supports the nerves.

b. Aloes-Sandalwood helps with bronchitis, Herpes, cystitis, urinary tract infections and skin tumors. It may be beneficial for acne, depression, pulmonary infections, menstrual problems, nervous tensions and dehydrated skin.

c. <u>For emotional clearing</u>: In ancient cultures, Aloes-Sandalwood was used medicinally to help relieve mental illness and heal the mind. Aloes-Sandalwood may unlock emotional trauma from the DNA of the cells, oxygenate the pineal and pituitary glands, thus improving overall attitude.

CASSIA - *Qadad* (Bow the Head)

Cassia oil is among the oldest known spices. Its Hebraic root is *qadad*, meaning to "bow the head in reverence." Is it any wonder that God mandated this spectacular oil be an ingredient in the holy anointing oil and the incense burned daily in the ancient Temple.

Cassia is an exotic and potent fragrance similar to vanilla-cinnamon, but distinctively unique in its chemical constituency. It is said that the women of Israel would bask in the fragrance of Cassia as the incense wafted through the Temple, and its enticing fragrance lingered upon them for days.

Cassia can be used as a sensual perfume, but with great care, as Cassia can easily burn sensitive skin. It may be diluted with olive oil for cosmetic and therapeutic purposes.

"All thy garments smell of Myrrh and Aloes and **Cassia,** out of the ivory palaces, whereby they have made thee glad." ~ *Psalm 45:8*

Essential Oil of Cassia is:

a. Anti-bacterial, anti-viral and anti-fungal. Cassia is one of the most antiseptic of oils and has been used by the British people specifically for flatulent dyspepsia or colic with nausea. The Chinese culture finds Cassia helpful for vascular disorders.

b. Cassia has been used historically to heal dry, sensitive skin when combined with highest grade mixing oils (*Recommend Young Living's V-6 Mixing Oil*).

c. For emotional clearing: When Cassia is diffused, it can help in the treatment of depression and stress-related conditions.

CYPRESS - *Tirzah* (Slender)

The Cypress Tree is known for strength and durability. The mighty Cypress groves of Lebanon were described in the **Apochryphal Book of Sirach** as *"trees which groweth up to the clouds."*

The Hebrew Scribe, Sirach, understood this when he wrote poetic references in praise of God's wisdom, comparing it to the magnetic power of essential oils:

34

*"Like a **Cedar** on Lebanon, ... like a **Cypress** on Mount Herman ...
Like **Cinnamon** or precious **Myrrh**...Like **Galbanum** and **Onycha**,
the odor of incense in the holy place..."* Sirach 24:13-17

The Hebraic root of Cypress is *tirzah*, meaning to "make slender." Some scholars believe that the "gopher wood" mentioned in the ***Torah*** as the material of which Noah built the Ark was actually a form of Cypress wood because of its durability under adverse conditions.

Essential Oil of Cypress is:

a. Supportive of the circulatory system; cypress oil supports the nerves and intestines. It is anti-infectious, anti-bacterial, anti-microbial, and strengthens blood capillaries. It is also great for use on teeth and gums.

b. Cypress is a good defense against arthritis, bronchitis, cramps, hemorrhoids, insomnia, intestinal parasites, menopausal symptoms, menstrual pain, pancreas insufficiencies, pulmonary infections, rheumatism, spasms, throat problems, varicose veins and fluid retention. Cypress has been found to have outstanding results when used in skin care, for lessening scar tissue and strengthening connective tissue.

c. <u>For emotional clearing</u>: Cypress influences, strengthens, and helps to ease the feeling of loss. It creates a sense of security, grounding and helps to heal emotional trauma.

*"He cuts down cedars for himself, and takes the **Cypress** and the Oak; He secures it for himself among the trees of the forest."*
~ *Isaiah 44:14*

In its prophetic sense, Cypress represents the Sanctuary of the Holy Feet of God in the coming Messianic Kingdom:

*"The **Cypress**, the Pine and the Box Tree together will beautify the Sanctuary ... where I will make the place of **My feet** glorious."*
~ *Isaiah 60:13*

ONYCHA -- *Shecheleth* (Aromatic Shell)
"Liquid Gold" from the Ancient Balsam Tree

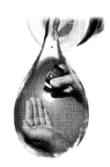

The Great Jewish Scholar *Rashi* claimed Onycha is a kind of root, while the *Talmud* suggests it came from an annual plant. Rabbi Gamaliel, the mentor of the Apostle Paul, says: "The balm of Onycha required for the incense exudes from the **Balsam** trees." (*P. Birbaum's Siddur Translation*)

Onycha's Hebraic root is sh^{e}cheleth, meaning an aromatic mussel or shell. D. Gary Young, N.D.'s research indicates that Onycha is extracted from Styrax benzoin, a type of resin, and was a part of the holy incense used in the Tabernacle in ancient Biblical times. (*Exodus 30:34*) Sirach, the author of Apochryphal writings, compared Onycha and other sweet spices to the unfathomable wisdom of *Adonai*. (*Sirach 24:15*)

Essential Oil of Onycha is:

a. Anti-inflammatory, antioxidant, antiseptic, carminative and expectorant. Helpful in combating arthritis, gout, asthma, bronchitis and skin conditions.

b. Onycha can be used for poor circulation, rheumatism, flu, chills, colic, coughs, laryngitis, cuts, chapped skin and inflamed and irritated skin.

c. <u>For emotional clearing</u>: Apply to 2nd Chakra to help overcome feelings of terror. *(Releasing Emotional Patterns, Dr. Mein)*

ROSE OF SHARON-CISTUS – *Chaba tstseleth* (Meadow Saffron)

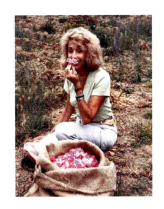

Cistus has a rich Biblical heritage; and in ancient times, it was collected from the hair of goats that browsed among the bushes. This rose-like flower is found in a fertile plain between Jaffa and Mount Carmel in Israel; and because this fertile plain is called *Sharon*, the Cistus is also called "Rose of Sharon."

Essential Oil of Rose of Sharon-Cistus is:

a. Anti-infectious, anti-viral, anti-bacterial; helps reduce inflammation; a powerful anti-hemorrhaging agent.

b. Helpful in combating bronchitis, respiratory infections, urinary tract infections, wounds and wrinkles. Effective with coughs, rhinitis and may strengthen the immune system. Rose of Sharon-Cistus has been studied for its therapeutic effect on cell regeneration.

c. <u>For emotional clearing</u>: Cistus helps express self-reliance for the Rescuer Archetype. *(Releasing Emotional Patterns With Essential Oils, Dr. Carolyn Mein)*

SPIKENARD - *Nard* (Earthy Fragrant Plant)

The Oil of Spikenard was transported to the Land of Israel all the way from the Himalayan Mountains in sealed alabaster boxes. Whenever a distinguished guest came to visit a Jewish home in Israel, the master or mistress of the house showed honor by breaking open the Spikenard and anointing the guest with fragrant oil. Both the Hebrew and the Roman cultures used Spikenard in their burial rituals. The Hebraic root of Spikenard is *Nard*, meaning an earthy aromatic plant.

Like Frankincense and Aloes-Sandalwood, Spikenard is 93% sesquiterpene in content and has the ability to bypass the blood-brain barrier.

Essential Oil of Spikenard is:

a. Anti-bacterial, anti-fungal, anti-inflammatory, and it creates a marvelous skin tonic.

b. Spikenard oil is known for helping in the treatment of allergic skin reactions. It also aids with candida, flatulent indigestion, insomnia, menstrual difficulties, migraine headaches, nausea, rashes, staph infections and tachycardia. Spikenard has been known to help in the healing of scar tissue.

c. According to Dr. Dietrich Gumbel, Spikenard strengthens the heart and circulatory system. *(Herbal Essence Therapy: Head, Upper Body And Lower)*

d. <u>For emotional clearing</u>: Spikenard is a relaxant (can make you sleepy) and is soothing to the mind.

In a prophetic sense, Oil of Spikenard helped to foretell the coming of the Messiah Yeshua. King Solomon penned the prophetic words 1,500 years before the Messiah came. The fulfillment of his prophecy is recorded in the Gospel of John, chapter 12, verses 2-3:

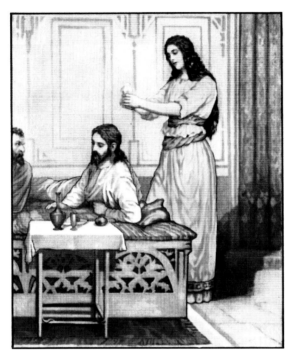

"While the king is at his table, my Oil of Spikenard sends forth its fragrance."
~ Song of Solomon 1:12

PINE – *Tid-Har* (Enduring, Lasting)

The legacy of the Pine has traveled from ancient Biblical times through today. Hippocrates, the father of western medicine, investigated Pine for its benefits to the respiratory system. Pine is used frequently for stressed muscles and joints and works well with the oil of *Eucalyptus Globulus*. Native Americans stuff their mattresses with pine needles to repel lice and fleas. Essential Oil of Pine has been used to treat lung infections and added to bath water to revitalize those suffering from mental and emotional fatigue.

*"I will plant in the wilderness...the oil tree, the cypress tree and the **Pine tree** ... together"* ~ Isaiah 41:19

*"The cypress, **the Pine** and the box tree together to beautify the place of my Sanctuary, the place of **my Feet** Glorious."*
~ Isaiah 60:13

Essential Oil of Pine is:

a. Hormone-like in its nature; Pine oil is anti-diabetic, cortisone-like in its constituents; antiseptic, lymphatic stimulant.

b. Pine is helpful when used for throat/lung/sinus infections; rheumatism/arthritis, skin parasites, urinary tract infection

c. <u>For emotional clearing</u>: Relieves anxiety and revitalizes the mind, body and spirit. Especially beneficial for feelings of unimportance. *(Releasing Emotional Patterns with Essential Oils ~ Dr. Carolyn Mein)*

FIR– *Ber-osh* (A Lance or Musical Instrument)

The rich, intoxicating fragrance of Fir entices thoughts of home and memories of happier times. In some traditional households, Fir is the fragrance of Christmas. In Biblical times, the Fir tree was the chosen material to carve and shape the instruments for worship in the Tabernacle.

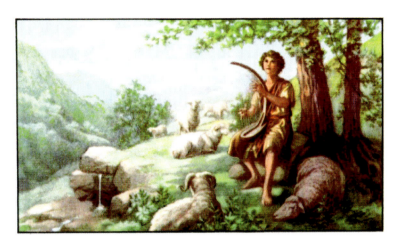

*"And King David and all the house of Israel played before the Lord on all manner of instruments made of **Fir** wood, even on harps and psalteries..."* ~ 2nd *Samuel 6:5*

Because of its highly prized essence and usage, chief architect Hiram chose the Fir tree for the building of King Solomon's Temple:

*"So Hiram gave Solomon Cedar and the timber of the **Fir** according to all that he desired."* ~ 1st *Kings 5:10*

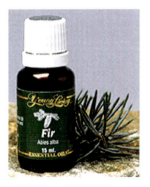

Essential Oil of Fir is:

a. Anti-fungal and helps to alleviate respiratory infections.

b. White Fir has an ORAC antioxidant rating of 47,900 and contains anti-tumoral properties.

c. <u>For emotional clearing</u>: White Fir is helpful with feelings of inadequacy (*Releasing Emotional Patterns with Essential Oils – Dr. Carolyn Mein*).

BALSAM FIR - *Tsor'iy* (Balm, Healing Ointment)

Whenever the word **"Balm"** appears in the Scriptures, it is the Hebrew word for **Balsam**. There is a 3,000 year-old Essential Oil distillery at *En Geddi*, discovered in the late 20th Century. This site is believed to be the location where Balsam Oil was distilled in ancient times.

With these new discoveries, many researchers now believe the legends from the *Frankincense Trail* (Oman to Petra) that the real Gold of that day was ***Liquid Gold***, e.g.: Balsam Oil, the "Balm of Gilead." Could it be that the *Magi* presented the Christ Child with three essential oils? **Frankincense, Myrrh** and **"Liquid" Gold**, the Oil of Balsam. *(Matthew 2:11)* The Greek word for Gold in this passage, *Chraomai*, literally means, **"to furnish what is needed."**

"...Take Balsam for her pain; perhaps she will be healed."
~ Jeremiah 51:8b

Essential Oil of Balsam Fir is:

a. An antioxidant. Its ORAC rating is 20,500 and contains the medical properties of an anti-coagulant and anti-inflammatory substance. Inhaling Balsam Fir may reduce the body's cortisol levels as much as 34%. *(D. Gary Young Seminar)*

b. Essential Oil of Balsam is for throat/lung/sinus infections; fatigue; arthritis/rheumatism, urinary tract infections, scoliosis, lumbago and sciatica.

c. <u>For emotional clearing</u>: Balsam Fir is helpful with feelings of inadequacy, separation, and of being scattered (*Releasing Emotional Patterns with Essential Oils, Dr. Carolyn Mein*). Balsam is for grounding, stimulating to the mind, and relaxing to the body.

CALAMUS – *Qaneh* (Measuring Reed or a Balance)

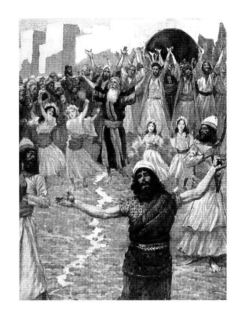

The Oil of Calamus, known in many regions as the Cane Oil, is extracted from the Root of the plant. It is used in Egypt to help improve mental focus, wisdom and sexuality. The Chinese use Calamus to aid in stroke recovery. Singers use Calamus oil to numb their throats so they can clear mucus and continue singing.

Essential Oil of Calamus is:

a. Beneficial to the digestive system, nervous complaints, headaches and may help to increase appetite.

b. Calamus can be used to reduce the desire for tobacco. When rubbed onto the feet, it helps eliminate foot odor. Helps also with asthma, bronchitis, colic, memory loss, stroke and depression.

c. <u>For emotional clearing</u>: Helps to bring genetically imprinted family patterns to the surface. Soothes intense emotions connected to dysfunctional family behavior. (*Vibrational Healing with Essential Oils -- Deborah Eidson*)

？ DID YOU KNOW

Therapeutic Grade Calamus Oil is found in Young Living's **Exodus II Biblical Blend (Code 3338)**?

The Law of the Tithe is a Universal Natural Law that when employed, will result in a 10-30-100-fold return. The Tithe is a powerful means to create abundance in your finances, your health, and your overall well-being. The Law of the Tithe is not reserved for religious devotees. As a Universal Law, it works for anyone who chooses to apply it. In Biblical times, the "Firstfruits of the Labors" were given as the Tithe. So the distillers of oils tithed Essential Oils.

"For you pay tithe of (pepper) **mint** and **anise** and **cumin**…"
~ *Matthew 23:23*

PEPPERMINT – *Heduosmon* (Gladness, Sweet Scent)

The Oil of Peppermint is a rich source of Menthol and has an ORAC antioxidant rating of 37,300. Peppermint is often used on the 6th *Chakra* of the Body's *Menorah* to enhance mental clarity. (Keep Oil Away from Eyes) Alan Hirsch, M.D. researched Peppermint to stimulate the brain's satiety center to curb appetite.

Essential Oil of Peppermint is:

a. Anti-inflammatory, anti-tumoral, anti-parasitic, anti-bacterial, anti-viral, anti-fungal. This oil opens blocked sinuses and stimulates the gallbladder and digestive system; a pain-reliever, and naturally quells fever in the body.

b. Other Uses For treating Rheumatism, Arthritis, respiratory infections, obesity, viral infections, Herpes, cold sores, fungal infections, Candida, headaches, nausea, skin conditions, varicose veins, scoliosis, lumbago, back problems.

c. <u>For emotional clearing</u>: Peppermint is supportive of releasing patterns of failure, fear of dependence, and restriction when applied directly to the Thymus gland *(Releasing Emotional Patterns with Essential Oils - Dr. Carolyn Mein).*

ANISE – *Anethon* (of the Dill)

The Oil of Anise is of the Parsley family and has an ORAC antioxidant rating of 3,337,000. With the distinctive scent of licorice, Anise is listed in Europe's first *Authoritative Guide to Medicines* as a treatment used more than 1,700 years ago. Historically, it was used for Whooping Cough and bronchitis.

Essential Oil of Anise is:

a. Supportive as a digestive stimulant, an anti-coagulant; an analgesic, antioxidant, diuretic; it is estrogen-like and anti-tumoral. Anise is useful in treating arthritis, rheumatism, cancer, colitis, bronchitis, flatulence, irritable bowel syndrome, parasites, menopause and PMS. Anise oil suppresses toxic convulsions induced by PTZ *(Pentylenetetrazole).* Reference *Supplement Research Updates – Ray Sahelian, M.D.*

b. <u>For emotional clearing</u>: Anise essential oil is emotionally balancing, dispels lethargy and helps the mind to focus. Good as a relaxant, with some beneficial effects to balance female hormones. Opens emotional blocks and recharges vital energy. Found in the Young Living Oil Blends *Awaken, Di-Gize* and *Dream Catcher.*

DID YOU KNOW…

The medicinal power of **Anise** *(Star of Anise)* is recognized as the plant source for the pharmaceutical drug ***Tamiflu***? *(Supplement Research Updates – Ray Sahelian, M.D.)*

CUMIN – *Kammon* (To Store Up, Preserve)

The Oil of Cumin is of the Parsley family and originates in Egypt. Cumin essential oil was used by the Hebrews as an antiseptic for circumcision and was retrieved from the tombs of the Egyptian Pharaohs. The Romans used it as a food preservative. Cumin's properties are anti-bacterial, anti-parasitic, antioxidant, antiseptic, antispasmodic, anti-viral, a digestive stimulant and an aphrodisiac. It has an ORAC antioxidant rating of 82,400.

Among the natural properties of Cumin is *Coumarin*. Coumarins are natural blood regulators. **Cumin essential oil should not be combined with the synthetic drug *Coumadin*.**

Essential Oil of Cumin is:

a. An immune stimulant and may help with poor circulation, wound healing and scars. This oil stimulates the appetite, supports digestion and acts as a liver regulator. Cumin is found in the Young Living Oil Blend, ***ImmuPower***. Cumin may have beneficial support for Diabetics as research suggests: *"Of a total sample of 1,039 **Diabetes Mellitus** subjects, the number of patients who actually used traditional remedies for treatment of diabetes was 313 (30.1%)… and the highest frequency (55.1% of patients) was for **Black Cumin**."* - ***E. Mediterranean Health Journal***

b. **Other Uses:** Traditionally, Cumin is one of the ingredients in *Curry* and helps with flatulence. When improperly digested toxic particles clog the channels in your Temple—including the intestines, lymphatic system, arteries and veins, capillaries, and genitourinary tract—alternative practitioners often use Cumin to release toxins.

MIRACLE OF EGYPTIAN GOLD

Legend tells us that the Children of Israel learned the art of the Apothecary during their 400 years of captivity in Egypt. Believing there is more truth in legend than written history, D. Gary Young created a unique and powerful blend of Biblical grade essential oils called **Egyptian Gold**. Every ingredient in the ***Egyptian Gold Oil Blend*** is mentioned throughout the pages of Scripture.

"And you shall take for yourself quality **Lavender,** *Myrrh, Cinnamon… and take pure Frankincense…"* ~ ***Exodus 30:23***

❓ DID YOU KNOW…

Lavender is mentioned in the Old Testament 25 times? The Hebrew word for **Lavender,** ***Bosem,*** appears in 25 Scripture verses. *(Strong's Exhaustive Concordance, #1314, and Webster's New World Hebrew Dictionary)*

Lavender was actually part of the Holy Anointing oil, which God commanded Moses to create for the Priests to apply in their Temple rituals. ***(Exodus 30:23)***

Egyptian Gold Oil Blend

Frankincense, Balsam Fir, Myrrh, Spikenard, Hyssop, Cedarwood, Rose, Cinnamon and Lavender Therapeutic Grade Essential Oils. For additional information on the ***Egyptian Gold Blend***, visit my website: **www.EssentialNews.com**

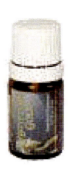

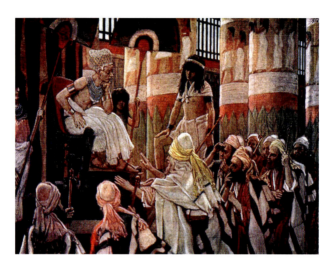

The Pomegranate And The Oils

Like the oil of Frankincense, the spiritual roots of the Pomegranate are legendary. When Moses was on Mount Sinai for his second 40-days and nights of instruction, it is believed he was given the instructions for building the Sanctuary and the Holy of Holies in the *Mishkan,* the Tabernacle in the Wilderness. These blueprints were later adapted for King Solomon's Temple.

Scriptural Essence tells us that a Pomegranate was to be sewn into the hem of the garment used by the High Priest. And later, Pomegranates were to be engraved around all the pillars that upheld the Temple. King Solomon accomplished it as a fulfillment of the prophecy.

In keeping with this pattern, our own bodies, **our Temples**, are greatly nourished when we infuse them with *the juice of the Pomegranate.*

"So he made the pillars and two rows of pomegranates above the network all around to cover the bands that were on top." ~ 1st Kings 7:17

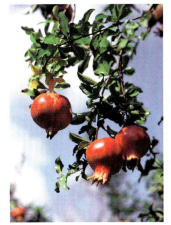

King Solomon captured the power and the value of the Pomegranate Juice in his Scriptural Love Song to the Shulamite woman:

"I would cause you to drink of spiced wine, of the juice of my pomegranate."
~ Song of Solomon 8:2

King Solomon also provided wisdom in combining the **Pomegranate Juice with Essential Oils**:

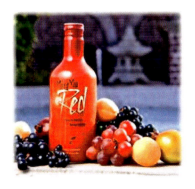

Ningxia Red
Pomegranate Juice

"Your Plants are an orchard of Pomegranates… fragrant henna with spikenard… calamus and cinnamon, with all the trees of frankincense, myrrh and aloes (sandalwood)."
~ Song of Solomon 4:13-14

I have found such an elixir which combines not only the power of **Pomegranate Juice** with the frequency of therapeutic grade **essential oils**, but also the **Berries** of Isaiah 17, 24 and James 3; the **Grape Seed** of Isaiah 24:13, and the **Apricot** considered in Jewish legend as the fruit of the Tree of Knowledge.

Additional information on this Scriptural Juice can be found at: **www.EssentialNews.com**

Proverbs 31
Virtuous Businesswoman

"There is Treasure to be Desired and Much <u>Oil</u>
in the House of the <u>Wise</u>."
~ Proverbs 21:20

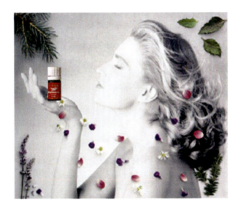

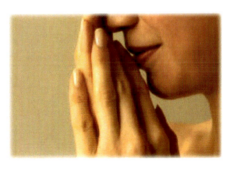

"A <u>Wise</u> Woman Builds Up Her House with Her <u>Hands</u>."
~ Proverbs 14:1

*"And now, my daughter, do not fear. I will do for you all that you request for all the people of my town know that you are a **virtuous** woman." – Ruth 3:11*

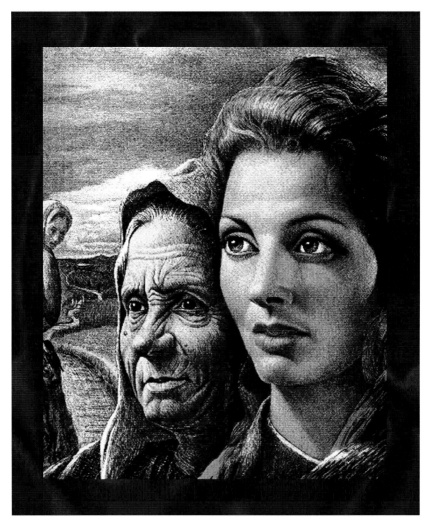

*"A **virtuous** woman is the crown to her husband..."*
~ Proverbs 12:4

The Virtuous Woman Experience

Proverbs 31 calls her a *"virtuous woman."* But in reality, the Hebrew word in Proverbs 31:10 is *chayil*. It means "**Powerful**; **Wealthy**; a **Force to be Reckoned With**" (*Strong's Exhaustive Concordance, #2428*). This Biblical Woman was a Woman of Divine Destiny — And so is every Woman of Faith!

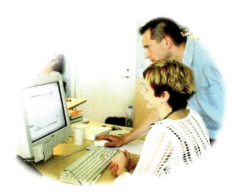

"The Heart of her Husband Safely Trusts in Her,
He has No Fear of Lack"
~ Proverbs 31:11

- o He is <u>not concerned</u> about money.
- o She is <u>earning an income from home</u>.
- o She is <u>not foolish</u> with her resources.

"She Does Him Good and Not Evil,
All the Days of Her Life."
~ Proverbs 31:12

She Ministers with Her Hands

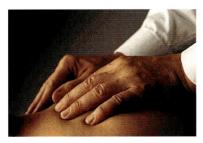

"She Willingly Works
with Her Hands."
~ Proverbs 31:13b

- o She is <u>diligent</u>
- o She <u>has a "hands-on" ministry</u>
- o She uses <u>Essential Oils</u>
- o She does this by "<u>Choice</u>"

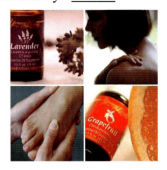

*"She stretches out her hand to her Tools,
and her Hand holds the Implement."
~ Proverbs 31:19*

She is Like a Merchant Ship

"She is like the Merchant Ships and Brings her Goods from Afar" – Proverbs 31:14

- o She is an <u>Entrepreneur</u>
- o She has a <u>Product</u>
- o She is <u>Open for Business</u>
- o She is <u>Profit-Oriented</u>
- o She makes <u>Independent</u> Decisions
- o She Goes Out and <u>Shares Her Gifts</u>

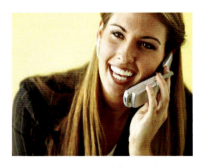

*"A Wise Woman Builds Up her House"
– Proverbs 14:1*

She Provides Food For Her Household

*"She Rises Early and Provides Food for her Household
and a Portion for her Partners"
~ Proverbs 31:14*

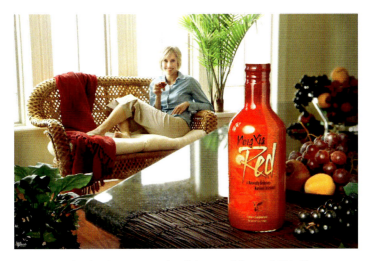

- She is Concerned with Health and Wellness
- She Gives Her Family Good Things to Eat
- She Educates Herself on Natural Health
- She Teaches her Partners To Do the Same
- She Builds Up her Partners

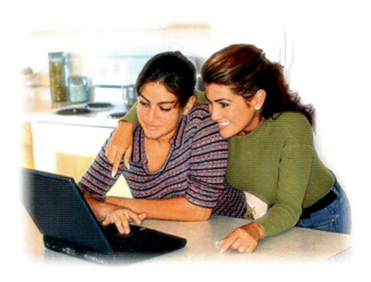

She is a Real Estate Investor

"She Considers a Field and Buys It; From Her Profits, She Plants a Vineyard."
~ Proverbs 31:16

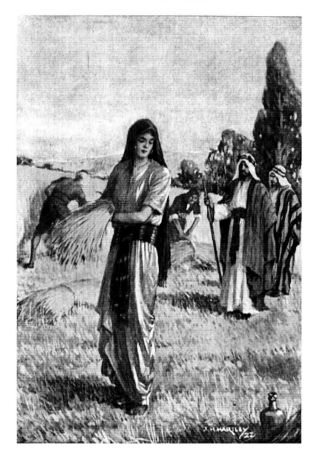

- o She Invests in Her Home-Based Business (e.g., She Plants Seeds in her Business)
- o She Invests in the Kingdom of God
- o She Invests in Her Family
- o She Invests in Oil (Essential)
- o She Invests in the Future
- o She Plans for Success
- o Her Cash Flow is More Than Sufficient

The Proverbs Woman is Strong

"She Girds Herself with Strength and Strengthens Her Arms."
~ Proverbs 31:17

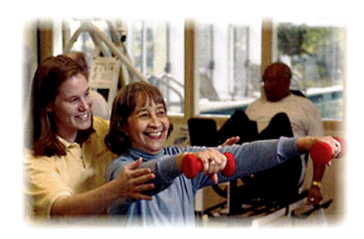

- o   She Maintains a Healthy Balance
- o   She Provides Nutritional Food for Her Family
- o   She Eats a Healthy Diet
- o   She Applies Essential Oils to Boost Her Immune System
- o   She Gives Her Body Rest
- o   She Exercises her Talents
- o   She Stays Strong Spiritually

Her Merchandise Is Good

"She Perceives that Her Merchandise is Good, and Her Lamp Does Not Go Out by Night."
~ Proverbs 31:18

- o   She knows the Value of her product
- o   She Confidently Sells it to Others
- o   She Believes in her Ability to Merchandise her Gifts
- o   She Believes that Others will Buy her product

Her Lamp Does Not Go Out By Night

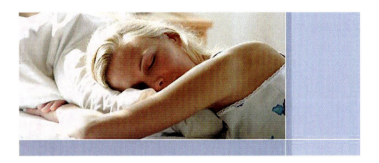

- o She <u>Earns</u> Money While She <u>Sleeps</u>
- o She <u>Leverages Her Time</u> and <u>Helps Others</u> do the Same
- o Her Business is Working <u>Around the Clock</u>

Her Business Complements Her Ministry

*"She Extends Her Hands to the Poor,
Yes She Reaches Out to the Needy."
~ Proverbs 31:20*

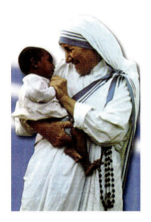

- o She's a <u>Friend</u> to those <u>Less Fortunate</u>
- o She <u>Gives Freely</u> to Those in Need
- o She <u>Encourages</u> Beginners to Succeed
- o She <u>Tithes</u> the Firstfruits of her Home-Based Business (Matt 23:23)

She Affords a Designer Wardrobe

"For All Her Household is Clothed with Scarlet, and She Makes Tapestry for Herself."
~ Proverbs 31:21-22

- o She Earns a <u>Healthy Income</u> from which she Buys Nice Things for Herself and Her family
- o She Knows and <u>Appreciates Value</u>
- o She Understands <u>Quality</u>
- o She Embraces her role as a Proverbs 31 Woman—To support her Family <u>FROM HOME</u>

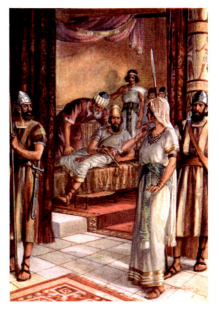

Her Husband Enjoys a Great Reputation

"Her Husband is Known in the Gates, When he sits Among the Elders of the Land."
~ Proverbs 31:21-23

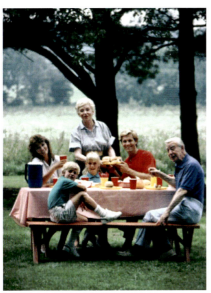

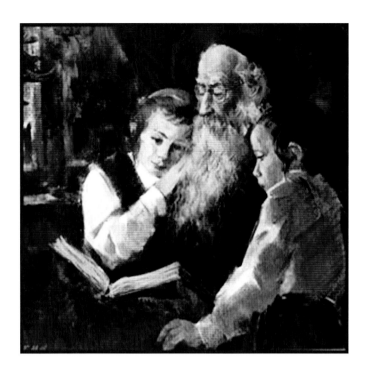

- o Her Husband has <u>Time Freedom</u>
- o Her Husband <u>Counsels</u> Young Men
- o Her Husband is <u>Not Stressed</u> About Finances
- o She Enables Him to be a <u>Leader</u>
- o Her Husband Follows his Calling and <u>Ministers to the Sick with Oils</u>, as was the Custom of Ancient Elders (James 5:14)

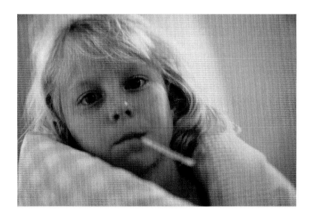

She Successfully Markets Her Product

*"She Makes Linen Garments and Sells Them
and Supplies Sachets for the Merchants."
~ Proverbs 31:21-24*

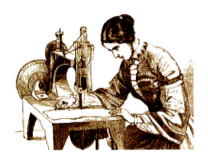

- Her <u>God-Given Talents</u> are Valued
- She Realizes the <u>Potential</u> of her Business
- She is a <u>Wise Negotiator</u>
- She Enjoys the <u>Continuing Growth and Success</u> of Her Home-Based Business

*"I have perceived that Nothing is Better than for a Woman to Rejoice
in Her own Works, for that is Her Heritage."
~ Ecclesiastes 3:22*

She is Watchful and Diligent

*"She Watches Over the Ways of her Household...."
~ Proverbs 31:27*

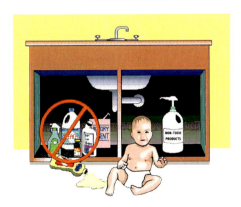

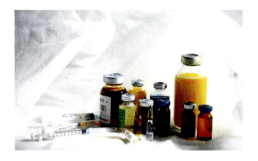

- o She is <u>Diligent in Learning</u> what is Best for her Family and Her Home
- o She Chooses Products that Will Not Harm Her Family—<u>She Reads Labels</u>
- o She Knows the <u>Dangers</u> of Processed and Re-Engineered Foods
- o She understands that Vaccines are man-made and that <u>God Gave Us</u> All-Natural Immune-Builders with <u>Essential Oils</u>

Visit Dr. Leonard Horowitz' website at <u>www.tetrahedron.org</u> for more information on Vaccines and Autism

Her Family Is Proud of Her

"Her Children Rise Up and Call Her Blessed;
Her Husband Praises Her."
~ Proverbs 31:28

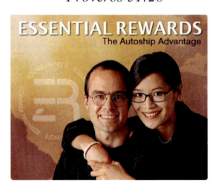

The Virtuous Woman is Successful in her <u>Home</u>, Her <u>Business</u>, Her <u>Family</u>, Her <u>Church</u>, Her <u>Community</u> and <u>Herself</u>.

⊙CBS NEWS

DATELINE—Washington March 24, 2005

"Lesley Stahl featured a group of highly educated women who had chosen to stay home full-time with their children. They recognized the benefit not only for their children but for themselves."

Her Own Works Will Praise Her

"Many Daughters Have Done Well…Give Them the Work of Their Hands and Let Their Own Works Praise Them in the Gates."
~ Proverbs 31:29-31

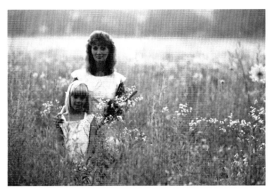

"The Older Women Shall <u>Counsel</u> the Younger Women to <u>Love</u> Their Husbands, to <u>Love</u> Their Children." ~ Titus 2:3-4

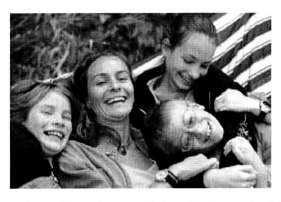

"Many Daughters have done well, but the Proverbs 31 Virtuous Woman Excels above them all."
~ Proverbs 31:29, Paraphrased

? DID YOU KNOW…

That the "Virtuous" Woman of Proverbs 31 is defined by the Poetic use of a Hebrew Acrostic? Beginning in verse 10 through verse 31 of the Proverb, you will find the entire Hebrew Alphabet *(Aleph-bet)* preceding the verses! It looks like this:

א – "Who can find a Virtuous Woman;"
ב – "The heart of her husband safely trusts;"
ג – "So he will have no lack of gain;"
ד – "She seeks wool and flax;"
ה – "She is like the merchant ships;"
ו – "She rises while it is still nighttime;"
ז – "She considers a field and buys it;"
ח – "She girds herself with strength;"
ט – "She perceives her Merchandise is good;"
י – "She stretches out her hand to her tools;"
כ – "She extends her hand to the poor;"
ל – "She is not afraid of snow for her household;"
מ – "She makes tapestry for herself;"
נ – "Her husband is known in the Gates;"
ס – "She makes linen garments and sells them;"
ע – "Strength and honor are her clothing;"
פ – "She opens her mouth with Wisdom;"
צ – "She watches over the ways of her household;"
ק – "She does not eat the bread of idleness;"
ר – "Her husband gives her praise;"
ש – "Charm is deceitful and beauty is passing;"
ת – "Give her the **Compensation** of her work, and let her own works praise her in the **Marketplace**."

❓ DID YOU ALSO KNOW…

That ancient Legend says Proverbs 31 was written by King Lemuel (King Solomon) as a tribute to his mother (Bathsheba). He is recalling how she taught him the Hebrew *Alphabet* as a child and also taught him what kind of Godly wife he should seek. **Lesson:** Solomon should have listened to his Mother!

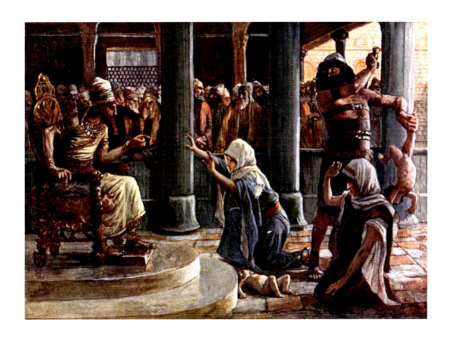

The Miracle of the Unseen Hand

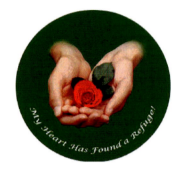

To some, this story will be almost unbelievable, and yet I know it's true because it happened to me. It all seems so amazing - it could be labeled a Science Fiction drama. Nevertheless, it is <u>fact</u>, and this is my account:

For nearly 40 years, I was plagued with the condition known as TMJ—Tempomandibular Joint Disease. My condition worsened over the years to the point at which I could barely open my mouth 20 percent of its capacity and no longer could sing the songs of the Psalmist, for which **Yeshua ha Mashiach** had anointed me.

By the fall of 2001, I sought expert health at the skilled and caring hands of Dr. Enrico Divito in Scottsdale, Arizona. I had heard of his success in treating TMJ with non-surgical methods. Medical tests, which included a full MRI, revealed that I suffered from Stage II and Stage III TMJ deterioration. And in the words of Dr. Randy Silberman, M.D., from the MRI Report, *"... There is apparent continuity of the joint effusions of the retrodiscal soft tissues, raising question of perforation;, and therefore, this could possibly be a Stage IV Internal Derangement...There is... bone marrow edema."* [swelling of fluid in the marrow.] *

Through the brilliant work of Dr. Divito, a full mouth splint was designed that provided a great measure of relief. But, it was necessary to wear the splint 24 hours a day, 7 days a week to maintain the stability. This meant that I could not sing, I could not teach, nor could I continue to do the Radio Interviews that help support my business.

* MRI Report, Biltmore Advanced Imaging Ctr. December 4, 2001

More than a year later, I decided to seek Yeshua, "**the God who Heals**" for a complete restoration of my jaw, though I must confess that my doubt and unbelief was very high. He led me to partake of the **"Grain Offering"** described in **Leviticus Chapter 2.** Since I had been involved with the essential oils of the Bible for 3 years, this particular Offering was compelling to me because it involved the use of Frankincense Oil.

After this, I was inspired to travel to Santa Monica, California to see a spiritually gifted friend, Mary Ervasti, who ministered with therapeutic grade essential oils as they relate to emotional trauma. Much research has been accomplished in this realm through the work of D. Gary Young, N.D., and Mary had trained under him.

Day 1 - Feb 16, 2003—the 14th of Adar 5763: *"The Jews celebrated the 14th day of Adar as a day of gladness and feasting, as a holiday and for sending gifts one to another."* **-- Esther 9:19**

As Mary anointed me with the proper oils, I experienced a birth trauma memory. As I released that memory, suddenly an *"unseen"* hand began to move my head and neck in motions similar to that of a chiropractor. Yet, according to Mary, no one was *physically* touching me. The adjustments went on for hours; and when they ceased, my $5,000 mouth splint no longer fit. But this was just the beginning…

Day 2 – **February 17th**, I returned to Phoenix, Arizona peacefully, knowing something had shifted in my face.

Day 3 - Feb 18th *"Chai,"* **the Day of Life** The Unseen Spiritual Hand returned, and movements and treatments increased in strength. I was in bed for 10 hours getting such energetically charged movements, that I was not able to leave the bed.

Day 4 - Feb 19th The miracle work continued with more intensity of movement. On this day there were strange movements within my sinuses. It felt as though a tiny Weaver was busy at work weaving a loom in the membranes of the sinus cavity. By the next morning, my breathing was deep and unencumbered as never before.

Over the next 12 months, the *Holy Spirit*, Whom I'd come to know as my Supernatural Chiropractor, worked diligently on my face, jaw, neck, head and spine. There were times when my physical body was moving in such bizarre positions, I still do not know to this day how it is that my neck didn't break. But with every adjustment, there was no pain, no bruising, swelling, no adverse response of any kind. Throughout the experience, I continued to use Frankincense and other healing oils from the Scriptures.

THE MIRACLES BEGIN

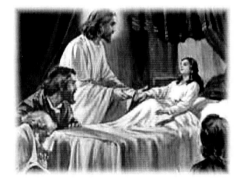

During the almost violent contortions and treatments, I often became exhausted. The sweet Spirit of Yeshua would then put me to sleep and do a quiet work on my jaw.

When I awakened, I was reminded of the story of Adam, when God put Adam to sleep to create the woman, Eve, from his rib. Since I was in bed for many hours every day, my home-based business was bound to suffer…And yet, it prospered. I continued to increase in rank and my commission checks grew. The Spirit whispered to me one day, *"**Will I not open the windows of Heaven and pour out a blessing?"** (Malachi 3:10b)*

On one occasion, when the power of His energy passing through me was very intense, an electrical blackout occurred in my neighborhood. It covered a six-block radius. No one in the neighborhood could explain it; and what's more, several of the automobile alarm systems went off at the same time. The owners were perplexed, as they were unable to disengage the alarm systems. In the midst of this chaos, my friend Mary Ervasti called me from California and asked, *"Janet, what's going on? My spirit is disquieted."* I said amazed, *"Mary, there's a major power outage here—even the phones are dead! How is it that you can call me?"* It was then I realized that the only phone in my home that worked was the one nearest my bed—the one on which Mary was speaking to me.

God allowed Mary's call to get through to pray with me. Mary suggested that the power outage was the result of the Holy Spirit rushing through my body at a very high frequency. There was no other explanation for her ability to call me on a "dead" phone. God permitted it; and after prayer, all car alarms ceased; the electricity returned to all houses; and the phones began to work again.

On another occasion, at 2 a.m. on a Sunday morning, the power of the Spirit was jerking me so violently, that I was thrust out of bed and onto my feet. Suddenly, all of the smoke alarms in my home went off simultaneously! It startled my husband and he rushed to find the source of the fire. He returned, saying, "I don't know why and I can't stop it!" I remembered to pray to Yeshua and the alarms instantly ceased.

Later that morning, my husband asked me to come to the front door to see something unexplainable. As we had just moved into a new home, the landscape was very immature. All of the flowers and bushes were in their infancy, no blooms and quite small. However, on that Sunday morning, I went to the door and opened it to find that all of the plants, flowers, trees in a straight line coming directly from my bed were in full bloom and maturity! The other half of the yard, however, that portion that remained outside of this supernatural energetic field was still covered with small, immature plants and <u>no blooms</u>.

I continued to pray, anoint myself with the healing oils of the Bible and experience the **Unseen Hand of Healing Energy.**

A week later, as the adjustments subsided for longer periods, I visited my hairdresser, Meredith Arnold, for my regular treatments. She tried 3 different times to put highlights in my hair as she had done for the past 2 years, but could not. As she put it, "***Your hair won't take any color—in fact, it doesn't even feel or look like real hair! There are literally gold strands running through your hair that have never been there before.***" *

The first photograph is a picture of the beautiful red and gold strands that permeated my hair during the height of the supernatural adjustments. The second photograph is my normal color and this returned after six weeks.

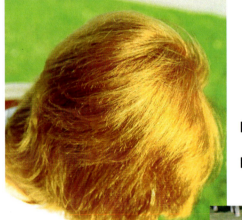

Left: Miracle Hair.

Below: Normal Hair.

* Meredith Arnold has retired from Cosmetology work, but has given her permission to quote her observation.

The Vision of War

March 29, 2003 –

It was 2 a.m. in the wee hours of the morning; I was in intensive Supernatural Treatments from ***the Unseen Hand***. Suddenly, the telephone rang and startled me. A call at 2 a.m. could only mean an emergency. But when I picked up the receiver, there was no response. I thought it must be the intense energy passing through my body that caused the phone to ring. Then I relaxed and fell asleep.

Next, I was keenly aware that I was experiencing a scene from the Middle East. The War in Iraq had recently begun. This vision was not like watching a movie screen, but I had the strongest impression of **"Being There."** I was an on-scene observer, watching a white car approaching my immediate area. The driver appeared to be Arab and was looking out his driver's side window. He was beckoning someone. Then I saw coming into my periphery, four American Soldiers in full uniform. They were closing in on the car. Suddenly, the driver pulled something up from his lap to the window and pointed it toward the soldier closest to the car.

A powerful white flash ensued and I awoke with a sense of panic! Later that morning, I turned on the radio and learned of the first homicide car bombing in the Iraq War. The details were chilling…It was as if the reporter experienced the same vision I had only hours before.

THE MIRACLE OF PSALMING

Because my healing was proceeding well, I found that I could once again sing and praise *Yeshua* in Psalms. And I had longed to experience again the miracle that occurred in 1995 when, at the bedside of a woman who had died, I sang in a Heavenly language under the frequency of the Holy Spirit. And suddenly, without warning or explanation, she was raised from the dead. Not only that, but the woman beside her in the Intensive Care Unit of Parkview Hospital in Fort Wayne, Indiana, who had been in a vegetative state was raised to full consciousness!

By the end of summer 2003, enough healing had taken place that I could freely sing psalms again. <u>This is my highest joy</u>. Yeshua inspired me in new ways to write psalms that have never been heard... psalms of healing tones and supernatural frequency. Not only was my TMJ reversing, but also Yeshua the Messiah was performing supernatural orthodontic measures.

The whole position of my bite and my teeth were shifting ever so gently. Spaces that were previously a part of my smile no longer existed. This enabled me to bite down more normally without the need for appliances.

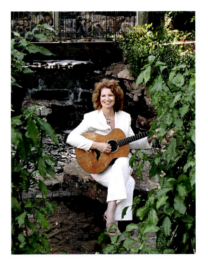

Today, my face appears different. The stress lines from the pain are no longer apparent. My smile is completely reshaped, more balanced, without one side of my mouth higher than the other. My jaw is restored and completely functional and my song is new and anointed with fresh oil.

"Trust in the Lord with your whole
  Heart and Mind and Soul and
Strength and He will direct your Path... and He will give you a New
  Song in the Night."
    Deut. 6:4; Proverbs 3:5-6;
      Psalm 42:8

A Final Thought…

The history of **Scriptural Essence** is rich with fragrance, romance, spirituality and miraculous healing. Only now in the 21st Century is the deeper understanding of what the Creator has given us to live life more abundantly being revealed. The **Ancient Temple Secrets** are more relevant than ever before, because the God of Heaven and Earth has ordained that you should…

"Walk In Health And Prosper, Even As Your Soul Prospers."
~ 3rd John 2

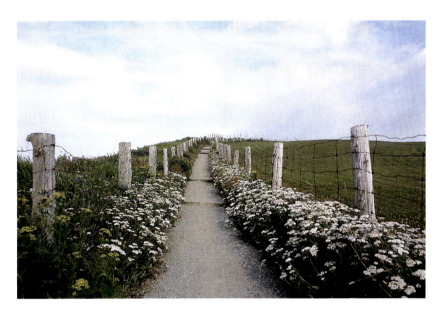

*The Path To Wellness
is Paved with Common Scents*

~ Janet McBride
Scriptural Essence

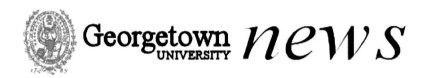

October 11, 2001

Oregano Oil May Protect Against Drug-Resistant Bacteria

"(Washington, DC) – Oil from the common herb oregano may be an effective treatment against dangerous, and sometimes drug-resistant bacteria, a Georgetown researcher has found. Two studies have shown that oregano oil—and, in particular, carvacrol, one of oregano's chemical components—appear to reduce infection as effectively as traditional antibiotics. These findings were presented at the American College of Nutrition's annual meeting October 6 and 7 in Orlando, Florida.

Harry G. Preuss, MD, MACN, CNS, professor of physiology and biophysics, and his research team, tested oregano oil on staphylococcus bacteria—which is responsible for a variety of severe infections and is becoming increasingly resistant to many antibiotics. The oregano oil at relatively low doses was found to inhibit the growth of staphylococcus bacteria in the test tubes as effectively as the standard antibiotics did." [Some researchers believe that Oregano is of the **Hyssop** Family, as constituents and similarities suggest.]

RUTGERS

December 6, 2001

FROM ANCIENT TRADITION TO 21ST CENTURY INDUSTRY
*Myrrh, Fragrant Resin With Ancient Heritage,
May Bear Anti-Cancer Agents*

NEW BRUNSWICK, NJ—Researchers have identified a compound in **Myrrh,** a bitter-tasting, fragrant resin has been used for thousands of years as an ointment, perfume, incense and embalming fluid, that they believe could be developed into a potent anticancer agent. The compound, which kills cancer cells in the laboratory, shows particular promise for the prevention and treatment of breast and prostate cancer, according to the researchers.

The finding is the first to identify an anticancer compound in myrrh, they say. It appears in the current (Nov. 26) print edition of the *Journal of Natural Products*, a peer-reviewed journal of the American Chemical Society, the world's largest scientific society. It was published in the Web version of the journal on Oct. 25.

"It's a very exciting discovery," says Mohamed M. Rafi, Ph.D., one of the co-researchers in the study and an assistant professor in the department of food science at Rutgers University in New Brunswick, New Jersey. "I'm optimistic that this compound can be developed into an anticancer drug," he says.

Ponce School Of Medicine
Department Of Pharmacology & Toxicology

By Jamie Matta, Ph.D.

July 16, 2003

Breast Cancer, DNA Repair And The Anti-Cancer Effects Of Young Living Frankincense Essential Oil

CLINICAL PROPERTIES OF FRANKINCENSE
- Anti-inflammatory and anti-arthritic activities in animals (Singh *et al.* 1986, Reddy *et al.* 1987).
- Blocks leukotriene synthesis by a potent inhibiting of 5-lipoxygenase; a key enzyme for the biosynthesis of leukotrienes (Safayhi et al. 1992). Leukotrienes are involved In the initiation and continuation of a variety of inflammatory diseases.
- Chronic inflammation is one of the risk factors for certain types of cancers.
- Pentacylic triterpenes have anti-proliferative and cytotoxic effects against different tumor types.

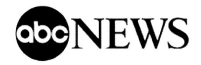

September 18, 2002

University of California-Davis

Aromatherapy Protects Against Disease

Researchers at the University of California-Davis have now released findings that suggest some smells, such as basil, rosemary, and cinnamon can actually protect the body against disease by acting as anti-oxidants - protective agents often found in fruits and vegetables. It is believed that anti-oxidants may reduce the risk of developing conditions such as cancer and heart disease by helping destroy free radicals, which are known to damage a cell's DNA.

In addition, a report this summer from the *Journal of Clinical Psychiatry* showed that aromatherapy with lemon balm oil has a significant calming effect for patients who are suffering from dementia. And though more research is needed, scientists are optimistic that more reports will follow.

There are many theories as to how aromatherapy works. Many advocates suggest that the scents trigger a "feel-good" effect in the brain. Aroma molecules may enter the part of the brain that is responsible for memory and emotion and induce emotional responses, which can immediately calm or energize the body.

Scriptural Essence

> To order additional copies of *Scriptural Essence* or to obtain the Biblical Oils, visit www.EssentialNews.com
>
> Call Janet McBride Toll Free at:
> 1-877-892-9688
> Email: virtualessence@cox.net